LIVING 40FIED

BUILDING MENTAL AND PHYSICAL RESILIENCE FOR MEN OVER 40:

STORIES OF PRACTICAL WISDOM

TAMAS FINTA

Copyright 40FIED 2024©

All rights reserved. No part of this guide may be reproduced in any form without permission in writing from the publisher, except in the case of brief quotations embodied in critical articles or reviews.

Dedication

This book is dedicated to my wife Emma for giving me her love and support in everything I do.

Acknowledgements

I owe tremendous gratitude to Melinda and Barnabas from Light Planning Media, whose creative ideas and professional filming and editing of interviews provided the essential source material for this book.

YouTube Channel Interviews

Check out my YouTube channel, where these stories were originally shared. The videos contain the same stories found in this book, along with additional footage created specifically for visual presentation. While this book contains the complete written narratives, the YouTube videos offer visual elements that complement the storytelling in a different format.

www.youtube.com/@40FIED

INTRODUCTION 5

LIVING FORTIFIED: THE AUTHOR'S JOURNEY 8

FINDING STRENGTH IN ADVERSITY: WITH EDEN LEE 28

THE WISDOM OF SIMPLICITY: A CONVERSATION WITH DAN JOHN 38

REDISCOVERING MOVEMENT: TIM ANDERSON'S ORIGINAL STRENGTH 57

THE IRON TAMER: BENDING STEEL AND SHAPING REALITY 73

STRENGTH BEYOND AGE: THE JOHN BROOKFIELD PHILOSOPHY 93

THE MIND-BODY CONNECTION WITH BILL LEE-EMERY 104

THE WAY OF DISCIPLINE: CAMERON QUINN'S MARTIAL ARTS JOURNEY 114

THE BEAST TAMER: SHAUN CAIRNS ON BUILDING STRENGTH THAT LASTS 130

EMBRACING DISCOMFORT: GEOFF WILSON'S JOURNEY INTO EXTRAORDINARY CHALLENGES 147

FINAL WORDS: THE ROAD AHEAD 168

INTRODUCTION

There's a moment in every man's life when he realises time is no longer just passing—it's leaving its mark. Perhaps it's when you can't quite keep up with your teenage son on the basketball court, or when recovering from a weekend project takes days instead of hours. Maybe it's simply catching your reflection and wondering when those gray hairs and laugh lines became so prominent.

If you're holding this book, chances are you've had that moment.

But here's what you might not realise yet: your forties, fifties, and beyond aren't just about managing decline—they can be the foundation for the most vibrant, strong, and fulfilling decades of your life. This isn't wishful thinking or empty motivation. It's the reality that countless men have discovered, and it's backed by science, expertise, and lived experience.

This book serves two essential purposes:

First, it offers you reliable, evidence-based knowledge from experts who have dedicated their lives to understanding the intricate connections between physical strength, health, and mental well-being. No fads, no miracle promises—just practical wisdom that works. These experts understand men's unique challenges as they age: shifting hormones, changing metabolism, increased responsibilities, and the psychological adjustments that come with middle age and beyond.

Second, and perhaps more importantly, these pages aim to inspire. To show you that prioritising your health isn't selfish—it's necessary. To demonstrate that making time for your wellbeing isn't a luxury—it's an investment that pays dividends in every area of your life. Through stories of men who've transformed their health, outlook, and lives after 40, you'll see possibilities rather than limitations.

Why does this matter? Because men over 40 are facing a health crisis that few are talking about. Our modern lifestyle wasn't designed for longevity or wellbeing. Our bodies were built to move, strain, and recover—not sit at desks for decades while stress hormones surge through our systems. Our minds were designed to solve immediate problems and find meaning—not to navigate endless digital distractions and economic pressures without a clear purpose.

The consequences are evident in rising rates of preventable disease, mental health struggles, and a pervasive sense of resignation that this is simply "what getting older feels like."

It doesn't have to be this way.

The men you'll meet in these pages—both experts and everyday individuals—have discovered something profound: that building strength, health, and wellbeing after 40 isn't about reclaiming youth. It's about claiming something new and potentially better: a powerful combination of physical capability, hard-earned wisdom, and purposeful living that is uniquely available to men in this stage of life. Whether you're already committed to your health or just beginning to consider making changes, whether you're looking to transform your life completely or simply make modest improvements, this book meets you where you are. The advice within these pages can be scaled and adapted to your specific circumstances, goals, and starting point.

As you turn these pages, I invite you to approach them not just as a reader, but as an active participant in your own story—one that isn't winding down, but entering a new and potentially remarkable chapter.

Your best years aren't behind you. They're still unfolding.

Let's begin.

LIVING FORTIFIED: THE AUTHOR'S JOURNEY

"You are braver than you believe, stronger than you seem, and smarter than you think."
-A.A.Milne

The seeds of my fitness journey were planted early. At just 8 years old, I found myself sweating through lap after lap on a 400-meter track in Budapest—not exactly what most kids picture when they think of table tennis. But this wasn't casual ping-pong. My dad's friend, who coached at a local club, had introduced me to the structured world of competitive training: three evenings a week plus Saturday mornings filled with fitness drills, agility exercises, and technical practice. While I loved the game, something told me this particular sport wouldn't be my life's calling.

Then I met someone who changed my trajectory. My best friend at school was a paradox—the strongest guy in our class, yet the quietest and calmest. At just 13, this jiujitsu practitioner carried himself with the discipline and composure of someone far older. What struck me most was how he never actually fought anyone. After just one demonstration of his abilities, nobody wanted to mess with him. That quiet confidence, that earned respect without aggression—I knew immediately I wanted that for myself.

So I began my martial arts journey at a local kung-fu school. There, amid the striking, kicking, grabbing, rolling, and balancing, I discovered something profound—a deep appreciation for the poetry of strength and movement. Between training sessions and weekend Bruce Lee and Jackie Chan movie marathons with my new training brothers, I was hooked. The physical training reshaped my body, but the psychological transformation ran deeper. In that kung-fu school, I learned respect, resilience, and camaraderie lessons. I learned to support those with less skill, to celebrate small improvements, and—perhaps most memorably—I learned punctuality the hard way.

The system was brutally simple: arrive late—even by a single second—and there was a protocol. You'd wait in the corner while everyone else began, then approach the assistant instructor and ask for your punishment or a "reminder," as we called it. Yes, ask for it. This wasn't mentioned in any brochure.

That requesting part was brilliant psychology. When you verbalise your own mistake, you own it. It transforms from feeling like an arbitrary injustice to personal responsibility. The punishment itself? Sometimes, just one other time, a series of low kicks to the outside of your thigh. If you've never experienced this, imagine a sharp and intense pain that makes it hard to remain standing afterward.

After receiving your "lesson," you'd limp to your spot and join practice as if nothing happened. This was 1980s Hungary—no one ran crying to their parents about "unfair treatment." It was simply how things were done. Looking back, those hard lessons built something valuable in me.

When I turned 18, our training shifted to more intensive sparring and fighting. Reality hit hard during these sessions when I noticed how much more a kick or punch hurt from bigger and heavier guys. Meanwhile, my strikes weren't hurting them as much as I hoped for. Physics was teaching me a lesson that my ego wasn't ready to accept: I needed more muscle mass.

Pumping Iron

Unlike in today's world, where gyms populate nearly every corner and shopping center, finding one back then required dedication. My solution was 40 minutes away via multiple bus lines, but that minor inconvenience wasn't stopping me. Of course, I approached it with all the patience a 19-year-old typically possesses—which is to say, absolutely none. My burning question, asked with complete seriousness: "Can I double my biceps size in six weeks?"

My scientific approach to strength development? Find the guy with the most impressive chest, arms, and shoulders, and copy everything he did. That was it—my entire methodology. The process relied entirely on experiential learning, without the benefit of expert guidance or corrective feedback. Despite all that, there was something magical about gyms in that era. No one wore headphones or stared at phones. People actually talked. We formed connections, shared advice, and celebrated improvements. Much like the martial arts school, the gym culture is centered around discipline and commitment.

According to the famous Swiss psychiatrist Carl Jung, life has four stages. The first one is the Athlete stage, in which we are primarily concerned with our body and how we look to others.

By trying things out, we develop our first insecurities. Slowly, we begin to recognise our strengths and weaknesses. We come into contact with our emotions and try to understand how they affect us. There is a constant need for acceptance and validation, and a complete absence of personal values and independent thinking. We mainly imitate others (parents, teachers, friends), having little room for autonomy. Adding a type of training that primarily focuses on aesthetics this time in my life was definitely about the way my body looked rather than about purpose or function.

Moving Down Under

Life sometimes delivers crossroads disguised as crises. In 2001, I lost my dad—a pivotal moment that forced me to confront some uncomfortable truths. Chief among them: my banking career was slowly suffocating my spirit. Sometimes it takes losing someone to realise you're also losing yourself.

My dad was only 54 when he passed away. I have vivid memories of my early childhood—him playing soccer with me and his friends, executing skillful moves and scoring goals while I watched with undisguised pride. He was the one who lifted me onto monkey bars, teaching me my first pull-ups, and who led our family on weekend hiking adventures through the Hungarian countryside.

But something changed around his mid-forties. The active man I admired gradually disappeared. He stopped moving. The soccer games ended. The hikes became memories. In their place came more cigarettes and more drinks. Then began the cycle of hospital visits that continued for years until his body finally surrendered.

After the initial wave of grief subsided, I found myself grappling with anger. Why hadn't he fought harder? Why hadn't he considered how his choices would affect my mother and me? Why hadn't he prioritised staying healthy and strong?

It took years to understand that depression had played a significant role in his decline—a revelation that transformed my understanding of health itself. I came to see that mental and physical well-being aren't separate domains but interdependent forces. One rarely flourishes while the other falters. Working on physical strength can lift mental fog; addressing emotional health often reawakens the desire for movement. The key is starting somewhere, anywhere—and understanding that seeking help isn't weakness but its opposite.

By 2002, with these insights still forming, I made a decision that shocked friends and family—I was moving to Australia. This wasn't just a change of scenery but a complete reinvention.

By this time, I had had 17 years of hard physical training under my belt, so I decided to complete my personal trainer certification. Soon after I got certified, I found myself in a whirlwind—racing between multiple gyms and health clubs, running group sessions and one-on-one training. The variety was intoxicating, the challenges constant. I had to rapidly develop an entirely new vocabulary—anatomy, exercise physiology, biomechanics—all in my second language. My financial English (full of terms like "quarterly projections" and "asset management") proved hilariously useless when trying to explain proper scapular retraction or hip hinge mechanics.

My Australian transformation reached its peak when I entered my first—and as it turned out, only—natural bodybuilding competition in Brisbane. Those 12 weeks of preparation redefined my understanding of discipline and willpower. Training 2-3 hours daily while following a diet so strict it made prison food look indulgent wasn't just physically demanding—it was a psychological gauntlet. My personality and body transformed, which my friends and family noted with a mixture of admiration and concern. "You're not you when you're hungry" takes on new meaning when you're surviving on measured chicken breast and broccoli for months on end. My fundamental objection to bodybuilding was, and remains, its disconnect from health, functional fitness, and mental well-being. The discipline fixates solely on aesthetics—competitors and judges alike value appearance above all else. No consideration is given to strength, movement quality, or physiological health markers. For these reasons, it ultimately wasn't the right pursuit for me.

I stood at the threshold between Jung's Athlete and Warrior archetypes, prepared to advance from physical mastery to a more purposeful chapter of life's journey. Nevertheless, I value having undertaken it as both a challenging test and an enriching experience.

Then came the humbling. Shortly after the competition, I encountered a strange object that would forever change my approach to fitness—a kettlebell. Looking at this cannonball with a handle, I was intrigued but not intimidated. After all, I was pressing 50kg dumbbells and leg-pressing 500kg! A 16kg or 24kg kettlebell seemed laughably light. "Let's see what this medieval-looking paperweight can do," I thought, signing up for a 2-day workshop with the cockiness of someone about to learn a painful lesson.

And painful it was. Kettlebell training demolished my bodybuilder's ego within the first hour. Unlike the predictable, controlled movements of machine-based training, a kettlebell becomes an extension of your body, revealing every flaw in your movement patterns with brutal honesty.

The problem wasn't strength—it was integration. My body, trained in isolation exercises while sitting or lying down, had no idea how to efficiently move an object through space with speed and power. That "lightweight" kettlebell found weaknesses I didn't know existed—limited mobility, poor stability, and dysfunctional movement patterns that no amount of mirror-muscle could hide.

After day one, I was so thoroughly humiliated and physically destroyed that I nearly skipped day two. Every fiber screamed in unfamiliar pain. But something deeper—perhaps that martial arts discipline—pushed me to return, making a silent promise to master this deceptively simple tool that had so thoroughly exposed my limitations.

The kettlebell doesn't sit in the middle of your palm like a bar or a dumbbell. Its centre of mass is off, outside your arm. Every second of kettlebell training, you have to control it. It never lets you rest completely. Unlike bodybuilding style training, where mainly the muscles you are targeting with the exercise work and the others can catch a break, kettlebell lifts require your entire muscle mass and nervous system to be active.

My fascination with kettlebells eventually took me across continents. I traveled to South Korea to complete my 3-day level 1 kettlebell instructor course, where I met Dave Whitley for the first time—a master whose skill and teaching would significantly influence my approach. Later, my pursuit of kettlebell mastery led me to Italy for my level 2 instructor certification, further deepening my understanding of this deceptively simple yet profoundly effective tool. I will never forget the graduation workout at the end of that course. Over 50 people were completing hundreds of kettlebell swings, squats, cleans, presses, and snatches while Master Instructor Fabio Zonin and his band blasted us with live hard rock. The energy and the atmosphere were on another level, with power exhaling and sound waves entering our bodies. My kind of party!

I should clarify that I'm not suggesting kettlebells are the only answer to strength training. Every method has its rightful place in the fitness universe. Machines provide a controlled environment perfect for beginners or rehabilitation. Barbells remain unmatched for developing maximal strength. Gymnastic bodyweight training builds incredible body control and pound-for-pound strength.

The key isn't which tool you choose, but finding what resonates with you—what you enjoy enough to practice consistently, what meets your specific needs, and what you'll stick with long enough to master and see its full potential. What definitely doesn't work is random exercises thrown together without a framework or coherent training plan. That approach leads nowhere except, potentially, to injury.

Let's Go Bush

"You know what would be fun?" is how conversations leading to terrible decisions often begin. In my case, it was clients suggesting I join them for something called the Oxfam 100—a casual little 100-kilometer trail walking/running race through the wilderness outside Melbourne. Having apparently learned nothing from the kettlebell humbling, I agreed with enthusiasm.

The event is a charity team challenge where Team #1 is traditionally reserved for Gurkhas from the British Army. If you're unfamiliar, Gurkhas are legendary soldiers recruited from the mountains of Nepal and North India—natural-born ultramarathoners who consider oxygen optional and gravity merely a suggestion. These warriors run the entire distance at a pace most mortals couldn't maintain on a treadmill with the incline set to "downhill."

Reality hit when we reached the 50-kilometer checkpoint, exhausted and feeling accomplished, only to learn the Gurkhas had already finished the entire race. But here's the beautiful realisation that came from that moment: their race wasn't our race. Our challenge wasn't about beating superhuman mountain warriors; it was about our preparation, limits, and victory. This philosophy crystallised into something I now share with all my clients: your training should never revolve around what others can lift or how fast others can move. The only meaningful comparison is between who you were yesterday and who you are today. You're walking your path; they're walking theirs—sometimes literally.

We completed the Oxfam in 22 hours, which included an unplanned 40-minute "rest" while medical staff treated me for hypothermia. Lesson painfully learned: respect the elements as much as the distance.

Yet despite this brush with the medical tent (or perhaps because of it), I fell in love with these endurance challenges. I went on to complete the 96km Kokoda Challenge in the Gold Coast Hinterland. Twice. There's something addictively transformative about these events that's hard to explain to those who haven't experienced them.

What I treasure most isn't crossing the finish line—it's the journey getting there. The preparation with teammates creates bonds forged through shared suffering and triumph. During the event itself, everyone eventually "hits the wall"—that moment when your body and mind simultaneously revolt against your life choices. It typically happens in the middle of the night, when you're following the narrow beam of your headlight, fighting sleep with each step. That's when the magic happens—you check on your mates, they check on you, share lollies or energy gels, and celebrate tiny milestones that seem ridiculous in any other context. "We made it to the next tree!" becomes a victory worth commemorating.

Talking about milestones. As a coach, I have found that not many people celebrate their milestones in their strength and fitness journey. As you go through the days and weeks of your training plan - provided that you had one to begin with - it is important that you stop for a moment and acknowledge when you accomplish something that was not in your reach at the start, however small the improvement might be. When they talk about how far they're from their goal, I often tell my clients that they also have to look at how far they have come. You should look at the gain instead of looking at the gap. It is a very human thing to do, but I see this mentality causes people to lose motivation and give up. It's only a little tweak of your perspective, and the whole journey looks very different.

During this time, I also opened my first private training studio and began the life of a small business owner.

One of the many rewards of running a fitness facility is the incredible people I've met—each with their own unique story and goals. I've been privileged to train clients for events ranging from military physicals to weddings, from ski trips to kettlebell instructor certifications. Some wanted to get bigger, others smaller. Some needed to build strength, others endurance, and many simply wanted to stop hurting.

As I crossed the threshold of 40 myself, I developed a deepening passion for helping people overcome pain and limitations—to reclaim activities they thought were lost to them forever. Few professional moments compare to the satisfaction of witnessing a client achieve their first pull-up or deadlift personal best. But the most profound rewards come in texts like: "Just finished the Inca Trail without knee pain!" or watching my client with Parkinson's get down on the floor and back up unassisted—achievements that transcend mere fitness.

This phase of my journey reflects what Jung called The Declaration Stage: The Age of Commitment. We integrate the wisdom and experience gathered from earlier stages at this juncture. We've gained clarity about what works for us and what doesn't, where we excel and where we struggle. We understand which pursuits are fruitful and which lead nowhere. We recognise what energises us and what depletes us. We've learned which relationships nourish us and which leave us diminished.

Simultaneously, we confront the realisation that our achievements and acquisitions haven't brought lasting fulfillment. We yearn to create meaningful impact. This drives us to articulate more clearly who we are and what purpose we serve. A profound desire to contribute emerges.

The things we once pursued relentlessly—wealth, influence, possessions—remain present in our lives but hold less sway over us. We've discovered that life encompasses so much more. We receive these blessings with gratitude but hold them lightly, ready to release them when necessary.

I also became a movement detective of sorts. Everywhere I went—grocery stores, parks, restaurants—I found myself observing how people moved. The ease or difficulty with which they performed simple actions. At my gym, I conducted movement assessments with new clients each week, and an unmistakable pattern emerged: people over 40 shared remarkably similar limitations.

Many struggled with fundamental movements: squatting comfortably, getting down to the floor and back up with fluidity, hanging from a bar, or simply standing on one leg. When I asked the more confident ones to try getting up from the floor without using their hands or with their legs crossed, most found it surprisingly challenging. These weren't isolated cases—they represented a widespread phenomenon.

This observation led to a critical insight: most people over 40 need a fundamentally different approach to fitness than 20-year-olds. Drawing on my accumulated knowledge from bodyweight training, kettlebells, barbell work, biomechanics, and gymnastics mobility, I developed a methodology specifically designed to address these common limitations, build strength without high injury risk, and fit efficiently into busy adult lives.

Let's pause to understand why injuries and pain occur in the first place. A framework I learned from Scott Sonnon's work has been particularly illuminating. Apart from trauma (falls, collisions, and other accidents), injuries typically stem from three primary causes:

Disuse: Not moving enough and not providing beneficial stress to the body to keep it resilient and mobile. Example: Not engaging in any form of physical activity. This often results in the loss and weakening of muscle tissue, deterioration of connective tissue (tendons and ligaments), and decreased range of motion. Simply put, use it or you'll lose it.

Misuse: Moving with dysfunction or performing exercises with poor form. Example: Playing recreational sports (golf, tennis, running) without addressing movement limitations and muscle weaknesses, which gradually breaks down tissues and results in pain.

Overuse: Excessive repetition, overtraining, or overdoing certain movements. Example: Physically demanding jobs requiring the same movements all day, such as a builder or a painter, office work where you operate a mouse with the same arm continuously, or overzealous, poorly designed exercise programs without adequate recovery.

Living Fortified

This journey has led me into what Jung called The Spirit Stage—a time when we begin to consider our broader impact and the value we create beyond our immediate achievements. It's not about winding down, but rather about expanding our perspective and finding new ways to contribute meaningfully.

In this stage, we start to recognise that we're far more than just the sum of our possessions, relationships, or accomplishments. There's a growing awareness of how our knowledge and experience can benefit others—not just today, but well into the future. We become more reflective about our priorities and more intentional about where we direct our energy and wisdom.

This isn't about mortality, but about possibilities—about creating something enduring while continuing to grow and evolve ourselves. It's about asking deeper questions and finding purpose in sharing what we've learned along the way.

A Debt of Gratitude

Any expertise I've gained over the years has come through a most generous form of education—one provided by the hundreds of clients who have trusted me with their bodies, their goals, and their vulnerabilities. Each person who walked through my door brought not just a specific challenge, but an opportunity for me to deepen my understanding.

The executive with mysterious shoulder pain that conventional approaches couldn't resolve. The veterinary surgeon who suffered from frequent back pain. The business owner who was considering giving up skiing due to knee pain. The teacher who had doubts about her upcoming bucket list hike of the Camino. The retired professional battling the effects of Parkinson's with quiet determination. Each presented puzzles that textbooks alone couldn't solve.

When standard protocols fell short, these clients' trust gave me the motivation to research further and apply evidence-based methods I had yet to explore. Their patience allowed me to pursue additional certifications and courses that expanded my toolkit. Their honest feedback—both when an approach worked brilliantly and when it needed adjustment—refined my application of these proven methods in ways no classroom could.

I've often told clients they were making progress, but the truth is they were simultaneously helping me progress. The diversity of bodies, histories, limitations, and goals I encountered created a living laboratory that demanded continuous learning. Without this rich variety of human experiences, I might have remained comfortable with a narrower set of skills and insights.

So while this book contains wisdom gathered from experts across the globe, its foundation was built session by session, challenge by challenge, with everyday people who simply wanted to move better, feel stronger, and live more fully. To all of you who allowed me to be part of your journey—thank you for being such an essential part of mine.

Embracing this Spirit Stage in my own journey, I've gradually stepped away from the day-to-day operations of the training facilities I built. My intimate studio nestled in the lush surroundings of Tamborine Mountain now thrives under Krisztina's stewardship. Her remarkable gift for identifying subtle movement dysfunctions and prescribing elegant, simple corrective exercises continues to transform clients' lives in ways that still amaze me.

Meanwhile, Club 40FIED in Arundel on the Gold Coast operates under my great friend and co-founder Jan's watchful eye. With decades of experience and an uncanny ability to draw forth hidden potential, Jan consistently proves to clients that their perceived limitations exist primarily in their minds. His coaching has guided countless individuals to achievements they once dismissed as impossible for themselves.

Seeing these talented professionals extend and enhance the work we began gives me profound satisfaction. Their success embodies the essence of this life stage—creating something that continues to serve others even as your own role evolves.

This transition in my professional life has allowed me to focus on the patterns I've observed throughout my career and pursue deeper solutions. The more I studied men over 40, the more obsessed I became with finding answers to their common challenges. My detective work evolved into a global quest—crossing three continents to track down ordinary experts and true pioneers. I sought out people who weren't just repeating conventional wisdom but were developing revolutionary approaches backed by science and proven through extraordinary results.

I interviewed coaches who were questioning established methods. I learned from practitioners who were helping seemingly "broken" bodies reclaim movements their owners thought were lost forever. I studied with practitioners who understood that a 40+ body isn't simply a degraded version of a younger one—it's a different ecosystem requiring a different and intelligent approach.

The knowledge gathered from these remarkable minds—combined with my own decades of trial, error, and observation—forms the foundation of my philosophy when it comes to training. I've distilled complex science into practical wisdom and translated cutting-edge research into actionable insights because I understand, deeply and completely, the challenges men face when starting—or restarting—their fitness journey in midlife. This understanding comes not just from research and observation, but from my own lived experience, feeling how my body tolerates the workload differently as I've gotten older.

This isn't about pursuing some impossible standard of youth or unrealistic physical perfection. It's about removing the limitations that prevent you from living fully. It's about building the strength, mobility, and resilience to embrace whatever challenges and adventures call to you.

I hope these pages provide not just information but transformation—simple, usable advice that enables you to live your most vital life. Because when you thrive physically, every area of your life improves. Your relationships deepen. Your work energises rather than depletes. Your capacity for joy expands.

The ripple effects extend far beyond you. By prioritising your health and wellbeing, you automatically enrich the lives of everyone around you. That's the true power of living fortified.

Reflection questions

1. Reflecting on Jung's life stages (The Athlete Stage focused on appearance and fitting in; The Warrior Stage centered on individuality and achievement; The Declaration Stage emphasising contribution and authentic purpose; The Spirit Stage concerned with legacy and wisdom), which do you identify with most strongly right now? How is that reflected in your approach to health and fitness?

2. Think about a physical limitation or challenge you currently face. How might shifting your perspective from "looking at the gap" to "looking at the gain" change your relationship with this challenge? What small improvements could you celebrate that you've been overlooking?

3. As you move through life's stages—from appearance-focused youth to achievement-oriented early adulthood, to purpose-driven midlife, and finally to legacy-concerned maturity—how have your priorities for physical training evolved? How might your current training approach better align with your life stage, personal values, and the activities that truly matter to you?

FINDING STRENGTH IN ADVERSITY: WITH EDEN LEE

The Dancer's Path

I'm sitting with Eden Lee in his Pilates studio, on Australia's Gold Coast. It's a bright, airy space with large windows that fill the room with natural light. Just weeks earlier, this same space hosted a Wim Hof Method workshop where I first met Eden and was struck by his unique perspective on movement, recovery, and the human capacity for adaptation.

At first glance, Eden's tall frame and graceful bearing hint at his background, but there's an unexpected quality to his movements – a careful, deliberate precision that suggests someone who has had to relearn the fundamentals of motion.

'Eden owns Pilates Central on the Gold Coast in Australia,' I explain to the camera. 'I got to talk to Eden during the Wim Hof workshop, and I found that a lot of the things that happened to him as a man, as a mover, and as a teacher would be a great story worth sharing with others.'

When I ask about his professional background, I find that Eden's journey begins in an unexpected place. 'I professionally started working as a ballet dancer,' he explains. 'Through that, I had lots of travel experiences and lots of movement experiences.'

Eden's background as a male ballet dancer who later became a Pilates instructor immediately distinguishes his journey from typical fitness narratives. While many trainers come from sports or bodybuilding backgrounds, Eden's foundation in the disciplined, artistic world of ballet provided him with a unique understanding of movement. As he explains, this wasn't a direct path but an evolution: 'I learned different movement techniques along the way and then transitioned into teaching Pilates.'

The timing proved fortuitous. 'It happened to be a good time in history. Pilates was just becoming very popular,' he recalls. But what drew him to this specific practice wasn't a trend or an opportunity, but personal necessity. 'I've been injured a lot as a dancer and mainly used movement to cure those issues. And then I realised it was a great way to help others with their physical problems.'

This experience – using movement as medicine – would become central to Eden's approach and philosophy. His journey from performer to teacher wasn't a planned career progression but an organic evolution shaped by his own physical challenges and the realisation that what had helped him could help others.

Against the Grain

When I ask about the major obstacles he's faced as both a man and a mover, Eden's response is immediate and candid: 'So many. Where to begin?'

His first challenge came with his initial choice to pursue ballet – not an easy path for a young man at a 'pretty tough school in Sydney'. The social pressure and gender expectations created immediate tension. 'I certainly didn't tell anyone that I was a ballet dancer for a long time,' Eden admits. 'Until slowly, some of my friends started to find out, and then they'd give me a hard time about it. I had a few confrontations with people about being a dancer.'

These external challenges were compounded by internal struggles that Eden, as a teenage boy, didn't yet understand. 'I didn't even realise as a teenage boy that I was very anxious and I'd flit in and out of depression as a result of that.'

In what would become a pattern throughout his life, Eden instinctively turned to movement as medicine for his mental health. 'I'd harness physical movement as a therapeutic outlet for anxiety and depression, channeling that restless energy into activities that elevate my mood and well-being,' he explains. 'I'm one of those people who, if I work hard, I feel better. And that lasts for a long time.'

Beyond the social and psychological challenges, Eden faced physical limitations in his chosen profession due to his body type. 'My height and long limbs created natural disadvantages for certain movements,' he explains. 'In ballet, particularly, having long levers makes many technical elements more challenging. Physics simply works against you.'

The professional world of ballet presented its own unique frustrations. 'Being a dancer, it's very subjective. You're reliant on the opinion of somebody else,' Eden explains. 'There's no right way to do it or a wrong way to do it. If the person hiring you likes the way you're doing it that day, you get the job. If they don't, you don't get the job.'

This subjective evaluation system eventually pushed Eden towards independence. 'That's why I chose self-employment,' he explains. 'When challenges emerge, they're entirely my responsibility to address. The burden of others' expectations was taking a genuine toll on my well-being.'

What emerges from Eden's reflections is a portrait of someone who has consistently chosen difficult paths – from ballet as a teenage boy to establishing his own movement studio – and has used the challenges along the way as catalysts for growth rather than reasons to retreat.

The Breaking Point

As our conversation continues, Eden reveals a physical challenge that dwarfs the others he's mentioned – a severe back injury that has defined much of his adult life.

'One of the biggest issues I had was with my spondylolisthesis, my back injury where I've had a little fracture and then the vertebrae shifted forward,' he explains. This wasn't a temporary setback but "an ongoing issue for the last 15 years or so."

Spondylolisthesis is a serious spinal condition where one vertebra slips forward over the bone below it, often compressing nerves and causing intense pain, weakness, and in severe cases, disability. For someone whose livelihood and identity are intimately connected to movement, this condition represents not just pain but an existential challenge. For Eden, the condition eventually necessitated surgical intervention.

'I had to go down the surgery path,' he says, 'and now I'm literally starting everything from baseline again.' At the time of our conversation, Eden is about five months post-operation, but his recovery has been far from smooth. 'The surgery went incredibly badly, so I'm really working from ground zero.'

Most people would view this situation with frustration or despair, but Eden's perspective reveals the philosophical core that has allowed him to navigate these challenges. 'In some ways, it's a great opportunity, finding all these things in myself again to reignite and fire up,' he reflects.

This ability to reframe adversity is not just positive thinking but a fundamental orientation toward life's challenges. 'I believe that within every bad moment, there are still opportunities to find a way forward and to push into finding out what it means to be you or a man or whatever, whatever that is.'

Eden's perspective perfectly aligns with Living Fortified's philosophy. 'What you've described is exactly what Fortified stands for,' I respond. 'The message is simple but powerful: difficulties aren't just obstacles—they're opportunities for growth. Instead of being broken by challenges, you can use them as momentum to push beyond your current limitations.'

This principle – finding growth within adversity – has not just been an abstract philosophy for Eden but a lived reality through some of his darkest moments.

Wisdom for the Middle Years

Given Eden's journey through physical setbacks and his expertise in movement, I'm curious about his advice for men over 40 who want to improve or maintain their physical condition.

His first words come with a humorous caution: 'Don't be like me and tear your bicep off trying to go too hard.' This reference to another injury he'd mentioned earlier emphasises his belief in the importance of proper guidance and realistic expectations.

'You want to get good information and build a plan going forward,' Eden advises. This measured approach runs counter to what he often observes in new clients. 'So often I see people come in. They're like, 'Okay, I want to come and see you five or six times a week. I want to do this, I want to do that, and I want to do it by yesterday.'

Instead, Eden advocates for sustainability and gradual progression. 'Really, you want to do something that one, you enjoy, and two, where you've got that sense of progression,' he explains. 'I'd prefer someone to come to me or you or anyone a couple of times a week and establish that as part of your routine and then just build on that so you get that positive flow.'

When it comes to specific exercises or modalities, Eden is refreshingly open-minded. 'In terms of what you actually physically do, I don't think it does matter,' he says. What matters more is finding the right guide and creating a sustainable routine. You want to find someone that you can work with, who you like working with, and somewhere you can go that is part of your routine, so you can get it. It's part of your life.'

Eden acknowledges the unique challenges of the middle years without surrendering to limiting beliefs. 'Forty plus is an interesting time, 'he observes. 'Not everything works the way it did when you're 25, and you've got to come to terms with that a little bit.'

However, he immediately balances this reality check with an emphasis on possibility. 'But also, you don't want to think, 'Okay, I'm old and broken, just give up,' he cautions. Looking at me, he adds, 'I see that you're in fantastic shape too. You want to maximise your potential, I think, is the way to go and just realise what that potential is.'

Eden concludes with an observation that encapsulates his optimistic yet realistic approach: "Most people's perception of what's possible after 40 is far more limited than what's actually available to you." That's really where we are, I think, in the world."

This perspective – acknowledging the realities of aging while rejecting arbitrary limitations – reflects Eden's broader philosophy of finding opportunities within constraints, a mindset that has served him well through physical challenges that would have sidelined many others.

The Art of Rebuilding

As our conversation draws to a close, what strikes me most about Eden's journey is his resilience and ability to find meaning and growth within severe physical limitations. His story offers a different kind of inspiration than the typical fitness narrative – not the uninterrupted ascent to peak performance, but the messy, non-linear process of rebuilding after significant setbacks.

Eden has had to relearn movement multiple times throughout his life – first as a ballet dancer working against the constraints of his natural build, then through various injuries, and now in the aftermath of complicated back surgery. Yet at each stage, he has approached the process not with resignation but with curiosity and presence.

His journey from ballet dancer to movement teacher has been shaped by these experiences, creating an approach that emphasises adaptation, mindfulness, and finding what works for the individual rather than forcing adherence to rigid systems. The breathwork and cold exposure practices that helped him navigate his most difficult periods have become integrated into his overall philosophy of movement and wellbeing.

Eden's story offers particularly valuable insights for men in midlife and beyond. His emphasis on consistency over intensity, enjoyment over obligation, and realistic progression over overnight transformation provides a sustainable template for physical development at any age. Most importantly, his lived experience demonstrates that even severe physical setbacks don't need to define one's capabilities or limit one's future potential.

As we say our goodbyes, I'm left reflecting on how Eden embodies the core message of the concept of Living Fortified – that through intelligent, consistent effort and the right mindset, men can continue to develop strength, mobility, and resilience well into middle age and beyond, even when the path includes significant obstacles. His journey reminds us that sometimes our greatest growth comes not from uninterrupted progress but from how we respond to the inevitable challenges along the way.

Reflection Questions

1. Reframing Adversity: Eden describes his catastrophic surgery outcome as "a great opportunity, finding all these things in myself again to reignite and fire up." Think about a significant setback in your own life—how might you reframe it as an opportunity for growth rather than just an obstacle? What hidden potential for development might exist within your current challenges?

2. The Present Moment as Refuge: Eden found that breath work and cold exposure provided crucial "cut through" moments that forced him to be present, offering relief from both physical pain and mental anguish. What practices or activities in your life bring you fully into the present moment? How might you expand these moments of presence to build greater resilience during difficult times?

3. Sustainable Progress vs. Quick Fixes: Eden observes that many people want dramatic results "by yesterday" rather than building sustainable routines. Where in your fitness journey or personal development have you prioritised intensity over consistency? How might adopting Eden's approach of "a couple of times a week and establish that as part of your routine" change your relationship with physical development at this stage of life?

THE WISDOM OF SIMPLICITY: A CONVERSATION WITH DAN JOHN

> *"Strength isn't just about lifting heavy things—it's about building a foundation that supports everything else in life."* - **Dan John**

On a pleasant, sunny morning in Salt Lake City, Utah, I'm sitting across from Dan John – strength coach, author, athlete, college professor, and, as he quickly adds with a grin, "grandfather, father, and crazy uncle." Dan has become something of a legend in the strength and conditioning world, known for his no-nonsense approach that strips away complexity and focuses on what actually works.

The Architecture of a Productive Life

When I ask Dan how he manages to balance his many responsibilities, his answer surprises me – he doesn't start his day in the morning. He starts it the night before.

"I think the key to a good day is preparation for a good night's sleep," Dan explains, leaning back in his chair. "My day starts around seven or eight o'clock at night. If you looked at my kitchen table upstairs, you'd see this little piece of paper where I write out my to-do list."

This simple habit – planning the next day before bed – is something Dan has been doing for years. He sets up the coffee pot so he wakes to the smell of brewing coffee, usually before his alarm even sounds. "Sometimes I'll look at my to-do list and think, 'Why don't I just do it right now?' So I'll send that email at 7 PM or handle whatever small tasks I can. Then when I roll out of bed the next morning, I can focus on what matters most."

Dan's morning routine is methodical. He tackles his college classes first, getting them "out of the way." Then comes any writing he needs to do – articles or books – while his mind is fresh. "For me, writing in the morning isn't a creative process. Writing in the morning is work. The creative stuff happens later in the day when I take a piece of paper and plan the next day's writing."

Perhaps most interesting is Dan's approach to eating. "I don't eat until I've gotten all my work done, until I've done my workout, and taken care of all the chores of the day. Then I eat." He explains this practice using a falconry term – "yarak" – which describes a state of heightened alertness and hunger that makes the bird more effective. Dan applies this same principle to himself, fueling his productivity with coffee and a bit of controlled hunger. "This is going to sound odd, but once I eat, my working part of the day is done. Sometimes I'm done by noon, and people say, 'You're done by noon?' Yeah, but I got up at five. I had a seven-hour day."

Dan's afternoons are where the magic happens. One day he might be throwing a javelin with a friend, another day taking his dog Sirius Black for a walk. Often, he's exploring solutions to problems he's observed in his gym. "I see my gym here like most people see a teaching hospital," he explains. "Teaching hospitals train doctors and nurses; I see my gym as a teaching gym."

Dan experiments when a client struggles with an exercise or a coach doesn't know how to teach a movement. "I'll go and play around with an exercise or an idea in the afternoon. Sometimes they fail miserably," he chuckles. "And sometimes they become the goblet squat. Sometimes they become the suitcase carry."

(It's important to note that the goblet squat, as we know it, was created by Dan John.)

Dan makes sure to keep his mind balanced, too. "I try to read something every day that's not part of my career," he says, gesturing to a well-worn copy of *The Count of Monte Cristo* on his shelf. "Just something to make sure I'm not constantly spiraling into just strength and conditioning and professional stuff."

Evenings are sacred – time for making dinner for his family, enjoying a glass of red wine on the back deck, and being present. "There is sometimes no separation between my work and my life because I love what I do. But I also have to ensure I'm here for my wife, daughters, grandchildren, and friends. If you have a brain like mine, that's a real concern." He circles back to where he started: "My typical day starts with the night before. It starts with preparation."

Finding Strength: Origins and Setbacks

When I ask Dan how his journey in fitness began, he thoughtfully reflects on a pivotal moment from 1965. "My aunt passed away,' he explains. 'We're an immigrant family, so "aunt" and "uncle" are relative terms – often no blood relations, but they're family. As I recall, she left us $500, and my brothers went to Sears and bought the Ted Williams barbell set – 110 pounds, about a 50-kilo set." Young Dan set himself a simple goal: to pick up the bar with the 10-pound plates on it. "I did it," he says with mock seriousness. "Drug-free." The barbell set came with a small instruction booklet that made a profound impression on him. "A couple of years ago, I found that booklet on eBay and bought it for $37, which was probably more than the original weightlifting set itself."

The straightforward cause-and-effect relationship captured Dan's imagination: "I fell in love with this idea that you could go into this thing, and if you worked on it, you got better at it. And if you continued coming back, you could add more weight and get better. It was all self-motivated, self-disciplined."

This early lesson has informed his entire life philosophy. "It's like with writing. People ask how I became a good writer. What did they think – that I was walking down the street one day and a lightning bolt hit me? No! You decide you want to write, and first you write a little bit, and it's not very good, but then you write more. Pretty soon, you have a thousand articles – some terrible, some pretty good. It's the process."

By the early 1970s, Dan's casual interest had evolved into something more serious when he wanted to play American football. He went to the library (which he jokingly explains to me is "a place where they have books") and found resources that would shape his approach to fitness. "They were very simple things: put the weights over your head, pick them up off the ground. Those were the basic workouts. Then they'd have a little mix of bodybuilding exercises after. But it was always putting the weights overhead and picking them up off the ground. Later on, when I got hurt, carry them."

Despite being the youngest and latest-blooming boy in his class, Dan found that his consistency with weights–training three days a week, while others might lift once a year, gave him an edge. "When finally my body decided to spring for puberty, I went boom, way past them. I just found that fascinating."

In Dan's life, there have been only a few periods when he couldn't lift – once after contracting a parasite in the Middle East that caused him to lose 40 pounds in two weeks, and another time when he hurt his back picking up a typewriter for a secretary. "That was a miserable time," he recalls. "I couldn't lift weights, so my doctor told me I should swim and learn to breathe bilaterally."

After that back injury, Dan's doctor prescribed alternative forms of movement. "I should swim and learn to bilateral breathe. Then I should go for walks and ride a bike. I figured swim, bike, walk, run – and I started doing these little sprint triathlons for about two years until my back came around."

Dan describes back pain with vivid imagery that anyone who's experienced it will recognise. "Backs are a funny thing. It's like getting hit by a lightning bolt when you hurt it. You're in pain for a year, and then one day you wake up and it's like an un-lightning bolt goes out of you. Where did that thing go?"

What happened next demonstrates a fascinating principle about the body's ability to remember strength. "When I was healed, I went back in the weight room and made the quickest progress I've ever made in my life. I was back to fairly high strength levels in a week. In two weeks, I started throwing the discus again, and it started going far." This recovery in 1987 coincided with meeting his wife, Tiffini, and kicked off what Dan calls the "second best period" of his athletic career. The first had been in the 1970s as a college athlete. Then, from 1987 to 1994, came another peak.

Years later, when his daughters were old enough, he started lifting with Tiffini because she wanted to learn Olympic lifting. Then catastrophe struck again. "I blew my wrist apart, and my career was over." But instead of quitting, Dan pivoted. "I started doing loaded carries, and then I had the best seasons of my life in my late 40s. At age 47 was the best year of my career as a discus thrower, and then ages 48, 49, and 50 were the best years of my Highland Games career."

Dan's eyes light up when I mention that some viewers might not be familiar with Highland Games. "You wear a kilt," he explains with a grin. "There are seven or nine events – you throw a heavy rock, you throw a bigger rock. There's the light weight for distance, the heavy weight for distance, the light hammer, the heavy hammer, and of course, the caber, which is the big log you'll see on the internet all the time."

Dan's accomplishments in this arena are impressive. "I won the largest Highland Games in the world, the Pleasanton Highland Games, two years in a row," he says. "Famously, I stepped in a hole turning the caber to win one year. One of the people said they heard a pop – and that's when I probably popped my hip out." He clarifies that it wasn't sports that ultimately damaged his hip. "Just for the record, I was born with a condition called pistol grip hips. My brother, my cousins, and my niece – we all have this same condition. Basically, you're going to have a total hip replacement the moment you're born."

Reflecting on his journey, Dan sums up five decades of consistency. "From 1965 to 2019, I've lifted weights three days a week almost the entire time."

The Pursuit of Longevity

Dan's voice softens when I ask what motivates him to keep training at 62. "It's going to be emotional for me," he warns, "but it is to dance at my granddaughter's wedding." He gestures to photos scattered around his home. "She's 5 years old now, so ideally 20 years from now." The timing of our interview is poignant. "You picked a tough day. Today's the 39th anniversary of my mother's death. Yesterday, my coach from junior college died. And in June, my brother died." He leans forward, his voice matter-of-fact but tinged with gravity. "My family doesn't live long. People always think I'm kidding at workshops, and I'm not. If we don't die in America's wars, we die young."

This harsh reality has shaped Dan's approach to health. "What I'm trying to do is all those little small things. I wear my seatbelt. I don't smoke. I drink water – you wouldn't notice it because I drink so much coffee, but I drink water. I eat vegetables. I see the dentist three times a year. I floss my teeth every day. I sleep soundly. I try to sleep eight or nine hours every night. I take time to breathe out and relax every day, have a glass of wine, and do what we're doing right here – talk. I try to maintain relationships."

Then comes the line that captures the essence of his motivation: "For me, going to the gym and training here is the only way I know that I can – sounds crazy – not die." I assure him it doesn't sound crazy at all.

"I just want... all I can do is what I can do," he continues. "If the angel of death is sitting right over there right now, then the angel of death is going to take me out today. But what I try to do is those small things that can help me be around a little while longer."

The competitive spirit that drove Dan as an athlete now fuels his approach to longevity. "I hate to call it a competition, but it is – I'm so competitive. For me, it's 'Okay, I'm going to run those numbers. I'm going to try to beat these numbers.'"

Dan recalls wisdom from his coach, Dick Notmeyer. "Dick told me one time in the gym, 'So Danny, what do you think's the secret to longevity?' When he asked a question, it usually meant 'Don't answer, I've got it for you.'" The answer was straightforward: "50 percent is DNA, 40 percent is probably lifestyle, and 10 percent is luck. You're driving down the freeway and someone texts, and you're out – that's bad luck. Or you bump into somebody on a plane and they tell you the secret to life and you follow it – that's good luck."

Though Dan's primary motivation is longevity, he admits there's a bit of vanity in the mix, too. "I don't think of myself necessarily as vain," he jokes, pointing to his face. "When you have a face like that, you don't have to worry about it!" But he shares a recent encounter that made his efforts feel worthwhile. "About a week ago, an Uber driver picked me up. We were talking, and she graduated from a local high school. I said, 'What year?' And she goes, 'Oh, way before you graduated from high school.' She was ten years younger than me and thought I was younger than her!" Dan's eyes crinkle at the corners as he laughs. "I thought to myself, that's worth three sets of eight. That's worth pushing the prowler. That's worth drinking water. That's worth rolling out of bed – to be 62 when someone thinks you're in your forties."

Dan's approach to health decisions is refreshingly pragmatic. "I always say cost-to-benefit ratios. Working out – here's the cost, but here's the benefit. The benefits might be huge for that extra 15, 20 minutes, half an hour of sleep. The idea is that it's all cost to benefit." He shares fascinating insights about small habits with outsized impacts. "I just read some interesting things recently about pressing the snooze button. It's such a small thing – my alarm clock goes off, and I reach over and press the snooze button, and I get ten more minutes of sleep. This article I read said, and I think it's true, that ten minutes of sleep just tells your brain you didn't have a good night's sleep. So you start your day with that extra ten minutes of sleep. It has a massive cost and almost no benefit."

Dan references a podcast featuring a female doctor discussing hormone health. "She said two things that made me go, 'That's true.' First, you need to go to bed within two hours of sundown for the rest of your life. Second, when you wake up, you should get up and start your day immediately without lingering in bed. Following these two principles can optimise your hormone profiles better than any supplement."

Living in Utah, Dan often follows this advice naturally. "I often go to bed at seven or eight at night. You go to bed within two hours of sundown, and you get up and go when you wake up. It might be the best thing you can do for your hormone profiles. Instead of popping a pill, those two things are probably better for you than all the nonsense we see online." This brings him back to the snooze button example.

"Something as simple as hitting the snooze button can undo all that. So it's cost-to-benefit – smoking costs are high, and the benefits are probably not very high. Drinking water is very inexpensive where I live, but the benefits are enormous."

The Path to Recovery and Growth

Dan describes a phenomenon he calls "toilet bowling" (with a humorous aside about the different directions toilets flush in our respective hemispheres). "Toilet bowling is when you stay up till midnight ten nights in a row, get up at six, and hit the snooze button. Because of your lack of sleep and hitting the snooze button, you don't get a good night's sleep."

The cascade effect continues: "Now you don't feel very good, so you drink a cup of coffee, but that's not enough. So you have a sugar rush by eating a bagel – and you might as well just take crack cocaine if you're going to eat empty carbs. In half an hour, you need something else, and you eat a candy bar. Then your insulin rush kicks in to balance that."

The long-term consequences are sobering. "What happens with many people is you begin to toilet bowl, and all of a sudden it's ten years later and your doctor says you're pre-diabetic or diabetic. Your knees, hips, and back hurt, and you've lost the spring in your spine as you walk. You start to lose your glutes."

When discussing how people can recover from years of neglected fitness, Dan references Dostoevsky's "The Brothers Karamazov," where a woman tells Father Zosima she lost her faith "bit by bit." His response? "Then you're going to have to get it back bit by bit." This philosophy perfectly captures Dan's approach to rebuilding physical health. When you've hit bottom—what he colorfully refers to as "the toilet bowl"—recovery happens through small, intentional changes:

"If you find yourself at the bottom of the toilet bowl," Dan explains, "recovery starts with simple changes. Tell yourself: 'I'm going to improve my sleep quality. I'm going to stop hitting the snooze button. I'm going to prepare for tomorrow before I go to bed.' For example, if you plan to eat breakfast, set it up in the slow cooker the night before so it's ready when you wake up."

These small changes compound quickly. Start with better sleep. Prepare healthy food the night before. Suddenly, you notice you're not craving that mid-morning candy bar. Bit by bit, you rebuild. The encouraging news? While poor habits might take a decade to fully develop, reversal happens much faster. "It took you ten years to get where you're at. It doesn't take ten years to get back," Dan insists. "In fact, weirdly, it seems—I hesitate to put an exact timeframe on it, but let's say ten weeks—you can turn your health around much faster than it took to decline in the first place."

For the typical 40+ person who hasn't exercised in decades—someone juggling a young family, mortgage payments, and long commutes—Dan offers a simple but powerful framework that avoids the biggest mistake most make: going too hard, too soon. "The biggest mistake you're going to make is with intensity and load thinking that you need to train like a Navy SEAL," he warns.

Instead, Dan advocates a three-pillar approach to rebuilding physical capacity. First is mobility, which he describes as "the free movement of the joints." His diagnostic tool is elegant in its simplicity: hang from a bar for 30 seconds. Most people struggle not because of grip strength but because their shoulders are too locked up to even get into position. The test reveals not just where you are, but what you need: "We need to open the joints up, literally open the joints up."

The second pillar is strategic muscle building, which isn't about vanity—it's about function and longevity. He focuses on three key areas, starting with the glutes. "Specifically in the areas of the glutes. You've got to get the glutes back online," he insists. "We're sitting on a goldmine right here. The butt reflects youth. If you've got a saggy butt, you might have six-pack abs and pecs and biceps, but when you walk down the beach, everyone just judges your age." Beyond aesthetics, he emphasizes: "Firm buttocks are the key to the fountain of youth. It's also, according to research, what most people look at. The opposite sex tends to look at the butt because that's an indicator of your fitness and your ability to reproduce."

The second focus area is what Dan calls "vertical work"—the muscles involved in overhead pushing and pulling. "We've got to get your shoulders back online. We've got to get your triceps back online." Third, core strength: "We've got to get your ab wall back online." With characteristic humor, he adds, "The best exercise is vomiting followed by laughing. But you've got to teach the ab wall to brace again."

The third pillar is walking. "I would much rather you walk than any other thing," Dan states emphatically. He references spine expert Dr. Stuart McGill's book "The Gift of Injury," which recommends 10-minute walks after every meal. What's particularly intriguing is Dan's observation that "three 10-minute walks seem to be better than a thirty-minute walk every day."

This approach confronts a fundamental flaw in how most people approach fitness. "The problem with the typical approach," Dan explains, "is that people spend 23½ hours a day being sedentary—sitting in chairs, lying in bed, watching TV, driving their car—and then expect that somehow, magically, a single 30-minute workout will fix everything. That's simply not realistic." The alternative—breaking movement into smaller, more frequent doses—creates a different relationship with physical activity. "You go sit, walk, sit, walk, sit, walk, and all of a sudden, things change."

What makes Dan's approach particularly insightful is how these elements work together. He describes mobility and hypertrophy as existing in a "yin-yang relationship": "As I mobilise my shoulder and build up and reawaken my deltoids, my shoulders, my upper back muscles, the triceps, and I do some mobility work, the two of them work together synergistically. If I stretch my hips and work my butt, my posture becomes better. The two are one. You can't really separate the two. And then walking brings the spring back."

Life Philosophy and Lasting Legacy

Dan's wisdom extends beyond sets and reps into life philosophy. He offers refreshingly practical advice about priorities at different stages of life: "I often say, guys, look, in your twenties or as a teenager, if you wanted to go to a music festival, sure, pump up your biceps. Great. In your forties, that might not be the most important muscle in your body. The glutes would be much more important. And your abs would be much more important."

For younger men fixated on appearance for social success, Dan's advice is both humorous and profound: "I always tell the guys in their twenties, when they say, 'I want to meet girls'... and I say, 'Man, if you learn how to talk like a human being and learn how to dance, you'd be miles better than working your abs and your biceps.'" With characteristic wit, he adds: "And I always joke, when I'm out and I have credit cards made out of carbon fiber, 'cause they're very high end. When I pull that card out, let me tell you, a lot of people at the table go, 'Whoa.' Learn how to talk like a human being and how to interact with people."

When asked about his greatest achievements, Dan reveals the values underpinning his approach to fitness and life. First, he mentions his children and his marriage. Then, he speaks to something broader: "My impact on the communities I'm involved with." Dan and his wife operate under a mission statement as elegantly simple as his fitness philosophy: "Make a Difference." He illustrates this with a recent example: "Just yesterday, one of my friends who is trying to go to the world championships and has a fundraiser, and I just sent him a bunch of money because that to me makes a difference."

In the academic realm, he points to his early writing on Beowulf with a touch of pride: "I wrote a thing on the Beowulf story back when I was young. And I still go back to that and I look at it and I go, that was pretty amazing." His books represent another source of satisfaction—not just for their commercial success, but for their impact. "Forty Years with a Whistle," he notes, "doesn't sell well, but I don't care." What matters more is that after Coach Lahati died, Skyline College uses that section of the book to talk about him: "What a tribute, to not only Coach Lahati, but to what I wrote." His book "Never Let Go" holds special significance, having "paid for both my daughter's educations." Some achievements transcend mere professional pride.

As an athlete, Dan cherishes moments when everything was on the line. At a Highland Games competition, facing an "impossible caber to turn," he found himself in a do-or-die situation. After his opponent's father prematurely celebrated victory, Dan describes what happened next: "I picked it up and I ran and I lost control. I stopped. I picked it up and I stopped again." On his third attempt with the 170-pound, 18-foot log, Dan achieved "Perfect 12. Win." Similarly, he recalls a football game where his preparation created a state of hyper-awareness: "When you can look at 11 people and know what they're about to do...the ball carrier would get the ball, and I would, I'd be right on him." During a national championship with a broken wrist, he faced another defining moment in weightlifting: "If I make the lift, I'm national champion. If I miss, it's not good." His wife Tiffini's colorful encouragement ("make the effen lift") helped push him through.

Dan reflects on these moments: "It's funny, two of the three are do-or-die situations. And I like that. I like do or die. I like that moment in sports and life where you step up or you don't. I love it."

Throughout his career, Dan has distilled his philosophy into a set of principles that apply to fitness and life beyond the gym. The first is to make a difference: "If you're on this earth, maybe for a reason, maybe not. I don't care. But you have a brain and you have resources. How can you leave this planet better than when you got here?" This principle extends from environmental stewardship to how we treat others, even to the simple act of cleaning up after yourself at the gym: "We should always leave the house cleaner than we found it."

The second is to maintain true balance. Dan emphasises balancing four key areas: "When I talk about work, when I talk about rest, when I talk about play, and the word pray, but I can also just mean alone time." This balance creates a positive spiral: "If I keep that balance, I can spiral out bigger and bigger. Take on more work. When I take on more work, I also have more fun."

Dan boils it down to fundamentals for physical training: "Pick weights up off the ground, put them up overhead, and carry them." His nutrition advice is refreshingly straightforward: "Drink water, eat veggies, eat protein." As he recounts, "At the Olympic Training Center years ago, the nutritionist said, 'I don't know what the big deal is, eat protein, eat veggies, and drink water. I don't know why everyone makes it a big deal.'"

Success principles aren't mysterious—they're simple but require consistent application. As discus thrower John Powell told Dan, "It was simple, not easy." Yet Dan challenges even this notion: "The secrets to life are very simple. But the funny thing is, I actually think they're also easy. Because once you do this right, sleep soundly, it becomes pretty easy to wake up, and fast, and drink water."

Good habits create momentum. When people ask how he manages to be a professor at two universities in different fields, his answer is straightforward: "I showed up on time to class and then I listened to my professors, and when they told me to do an assignment, I did it. And I always turn it in early to get feedback... and it just spirals."

His final principle came from Coach Ralph Maughan, who advised young Dan: "The secret to throwing the discus? You need to lift weights three days a week, throw the discus four days a week, for the next eight years." As Dan notes, "Most people miss the eight-year part. Everyone wants to do it in one year." Coach Maughan's further wisdom sealed Dan's approach to athletic development: "The secret to being a great track athlete is little and often over the long haul... As a division one athlete, you need to make yourself a slave to good habits."

These principles—making a difference, maintaining balance, embracing simplicity, and being consistent—form the core of Dan John's approach. They offer a roadmap not just to physical development, but to a life well-lived.

Reflection Questions

1. Intentional Preparation: Dan John begins his day the night before, setting up his tomorrow with deliberate planning. How might reframing your day to start with evening preparation rather than morning routines transform your productivity and peace of mind? What small, concrete changes could you implement tonight?

2. The Cost-Benefit Philosophy: Throughout the interview, Dan evaluates habits through a cost-to-benefit lens—from the snooze button's hidden costs to the outsized benefits of consistent movement. What three daily habits in your life deserve reevaluation under this framework? Which have high costs with minimal returns and offer significant benefits you might be undervaluing?

3. Making a Difference: Dan operates under the simple mission statement: "Make a Difference." If you were to honestly assess your impact on the communities you inhabit—family, work, neighborhood, greater community—where are you currently making the most meaningful difference, and where do you see untapped potential to leave things "better than you found them"?

REDISCOVERING MOVEMENT: TIM ANDERSON'S ORIGINAL STRENGTH

"You are not supposed to be weak or fragile. Refuse to accept these conditions. Move and heal." **- Tim Anderson**

The Reset Button

I am visiting the quiet town of Fuquay-Varina, North Carolina, to meet with Tim Anderson, a former firefighter, movement specialist, and founder of Original Strength Institute. Around us, the training studio is refreshingly minimalist – no rows of gleaming machines or walls of heavy weights, just open space designed for human bodies to move as they were meant to.

"So what is Original Strength Institute?" I ask, opening our conversation.

Tim's answer is deceptively simple: "We are an independent private training studio or group training studio where we simply remind people how they were designed to move so that they can become stronger and healthier and live their life the way they want to."

This straightforward mission statement belies a revolutionary approach to fitness that has drawn people from around the world to learn from Tim. His method challenges conventional wisdom about exercise, focusing not on muscle isolation or complex training protocols but on rediscovering the foundational movements we all naturally mastered as children.

When I ask about his background, Tim's journey reveals itself as both ordinary and extraordinary. Born and raised in this small North Carolina town, he worked as a professional firefighter while moonlighting as a personal trainer. But it was his own physical struggles that led to his breakthrough approach.

"I got some overuse injuries," he explains, "and I was looking for corrective exercises to not hurt anymore." With characteristic self-deprecation, he adds, "'Cause I was too stupid to just stop doing what I was doing."

As many men in their forties might recognise, Tim's initial response to pain wasn't to rest but to push through. The corrective exercises he found weren't working because he wasn't addressing the root cause. It was at this point of frustration that Tim took an unusual approach.

"I just wanted to figure out how to train to be bulletproof because I like Superman and I wanted to be Superman," he says with a disarming smile. "And I started to look at the way a child moves."

This revelation – that the movement patterns we naturally develop as infants and toddlers might hold the key to restoring adult bodies – became the foundation of Original Strength. "We're all designed to be strong and healthy, and we all still have this same movement template that a child has," Tim explains. "So you can press reset on your body and get your strength, health, mobility, and life back."

The concept caught on so powerfully that Tim eventually left firefighting to devote himself full-time to teaching people how to reconnect with their natural movement patterns. "This was way too much fun to continue doing that," he says of the career change.

The Developmental Blueprint

Tim elaborates on the central insight that drives his approach as our conversation deepens. "A child is born with a developmental sequence," he explains. "It's like a program, a series of programs that's designed to make the child strong without anybody teaching the child how to do it."

This innate programming allows infants to progress from helplessness to walking and running without formal instruction. "Very few babies can afford to pay personal trainers," Tim jokes, highlighting the remarkable fact that our bodies naturally know how to develop strength and coordination.

The Original Strength system focuses on reactivating this developmental sequence through five primary movements: diaphragmatic breathing, head control, rolling, rocking, and crawling. "Those are the movements that we are all designed to do," Tim says. "And those are the movements that we remind people how to do to restore their strength."

While these movements might seem elementary compared to complex exercise routines, Tim emphasises their profound impact: "We try to change the paradigm of what health and strength is or how you're supposed to get there."

This paradigm shift involves recognising that strength isn't something external to acquire but rather an inherent capacity to reclaim. "We're really telling them that they are strong," Tim says. "They may not realise that they're strong, but they have everything in their body that they need to be strong."

This perspective is revolutionary for many men over forty who have spent decades trying to build strength through grueling workouts or chasing fitness trends. "We really try to erase the idea of exercise," Tim explains, challenging conventional wisdom about what physical training should look like. "It doesn't have to hurt. It doesn't have to be ridiculously hard... simple is oftentimes the best route to get anywhere."

He illustrates this with a straightforward analogy: 'If you and I want to get from point A to point B, we'll arrive much faster by taking a direct path rather than meandering around. When our goal is simply to reach our destination, we should focus on going straight there.'"

The Memory Trap

When I ask about common issues he sees in men over forty, Tim identifies two primary challenges. "The most common thing we see here or anywhere probably is breathing," he notes. "Most people, especially guys, because we want to be big chested, want to look strong, we learned how to breathe up here", tapping at his chest, "so we forget how to breathe down here." pointing at his stomach. "But strength is down here at the belly and not at the chest."

This observation – that many men have lost the natural diaphragmatic breathing pattern of infants in favour of shallow chest breathing – points to a fundamental disconnect from our bodies' optimal functioning.

Tim's second major issue resonates with many midlife men: "They know they want to get in shape or feel better, but they're operating off of their memory for how they may have done it when they were 18, 15, or 16."

This memory trap leads to a predictable sequence of events: "They go from being, say, 45 to gonna get back in shape. And they jump back into what they did when they were 17. And they jumped in way too deep. Their body wasn't young, soft, and pliable like it was back then. And they're operating off their memory, so they do something that was too advanced for their body after years of inactivity, and they end up hurting themselves."

The consequences of this approach extend beyond immediate injury. Tim observes that many men don't account for the accumulated life experience in their bodies: "If you're in your mid-40s, you've got at least 20 to 25 years' worth of history built up in your body that you never had when you were a teenager. You didn't have any history built up in your body yet. You were still a spring chicken."

This history – the accumulated stresses, injuries, adaptations, and compensations – means that returning to fitness requires a different approach than the one that worked in youth. Family responsibilities, career demands, and decades of physical patterns have created a body that needs restoration before it can handle intense training.

The Dog Bite Incident

Our serious conversation takes a humorous turn when I mention Dan John, the strength coach I'd recently interviewed in Salt Lake City. Tim's face lights up as he recalls staying at Dan's house and an unexpected encounter with Dan's dog, Sirius Black.

"Dan John is my friend, and I love Dan John," Tim begins, "and Dan John talks really fast, so I'm gonna try to talk like Dan John." His impression of the renowned coach brings laughter to the room.

While staying at Dan John's house, Tim was accused of being overly tactile with household items—a charge he playfully denies. 'I didn't touch anything, Dan,' Tim insists with feigned innocence, before adding the punchline: 'Except your dog.'"

Tim then explains that he was doing one of his daily movement practices – standing cross crawls, where you touch opposite elbow to knee – when Dan's dog had an unexpected reaction.

"It turns out if you do cross crawls in front of Sirius Black, the dog freaks out," Tim says, shaking his head. "So I'm standing there doing cross crawls, and the freaking dog bites me in the butt! I'm like, what the heck?"

The incident didn't end there. "I didn't learn the first time, but figured out the pattern. Every time I did cross crawls, the dog would start running, sneak up behind me, and bite."

This anecdote, told with Tim's characteristic good humor, illustrates his commitment to daily movement practice – even when visiting friends and risking canine disapproval. It's a testament to his belief that consistent, simple movements are the foundation of lasting physical well-being.

Measure What Matters

As our conversation turns to practical implementation, Tim offers insight into how he structures training for himself and his clients. Rather than focusing solely on weight lifted or reps completed, he emphasises time under task as a primary metric.

"I like to do things in blocks of time," he explains, "because I'm trying to develop work capacity, which in my mind is the way to take the breaks and limits off the body."

His approach involves setting a target for accumulated work time – often ten minutes – and then measuring how long it takes to complete that work with necessary rest periods. "If I aim to crawl for 10 minutes of work, I have two watches. I have the one watch I start when I get started, and I crawl until I have to stop, and then I stop that time. But the other watch is still accumulating actual time."

This dual timekeeping creates a precise measurement of capacity: "It may have taken me an actual 45 minutes to crawl 10 minutes' worth of work. That's great, because now I have a parameter. I have measurements. I have data."

The beauty of this approach is that progress becomes unmistakable. "Three weeks from now, if I crawl for 10 minutes of work, but I do it in 22 minutes, well, I know that I have doubled my ability to do that task."

As capacity increases, the gap between work time and elapsed time narrows: "Four weeks from then, if I can crawl for 10 minutes of work in 12 minutes, well, I'm a lot stronger, and I'm a lot more efficient, and I know I'm moving better. And then, five days later, when I can crawl for 10 minutes in 10 minutes, I can do anything. I can do anything I want to do."

This methodology provides both objective feedback and psychological reinforcement. "If you don't know where you started, you don't know when you get to wherever you want to be," Tim notes. The approach works with any challenging movement – carries, squats, pushups – as long as there's a way to measure accumulated work time against elapsed time.

To put this into perspective, I was given the chance to try Tim's five-minute crawling test, a standard challenge for all his clients. The knees aren't touching the floor; therefore, you have to deal with your whole body weight and fight gravity. Fortunately, I'd been incorporating crawling into my workouts, so I managed it. Still, let me tell you, five minutes feels like an eternity when you're crawling on your hands and toes.

The Crawling Revolution

Tim's reputation in the fitness world has been significantly shaped by his advocacy for crawling as a fundamental movement pattern. His one-mile Spider-Man crawl video became something of a legend in movement circles. When I mention this, Tim smiles, acknowledging his reputation as "the crazy dude that crawls forever."

I ask him to explain the significance of this seemingly simple movement. "Crawling is an amazing movement," he says with genuine enthusiasm. "Matter of fact, we were all programmed to crawl, and that is the movement that was designed to get us strong enough to be on two feet and to conquer the world."

The power of crawling extends beyond its developmental role: "It's also the foundation of our gait pattern... your gait pattern keeps you strong and healthy, which means walking keeps you strong and healthy, if you walk right. How do you know if you walk right? You crawl."

Tim explains that crawling creates demands the body doesn't encounter in normal walking: "Crawling is also harder. It's not as efficient as walking. And it requires all four limbs to move together in a rhythmic, coordinated fashion."

This coordination has ripple effects throughout the entire system: "It really ties your body together very, very well. It makes all your muscles do their job. It teaches your body where everything's at... It strengthens your nervous system. It's like a fountain of youth, really. It turns back the clock."

I thought about the "crawling to be bulletproof test" he made me do earlier. "I need a huge breakfast after that test," I admit. "It's a lot harder than it looks."

Tim nods knowingly: "I will tell you this one secret about crawling. It's a great way to make hard things very easy. No matter what they are. Because once crawling becomes easy, everything's easy."

The Foundation Movements

As our time together draws to a close, I ask Tim to identify the three most impactful movements for someone looking to reclaim their physical capacity. His response is characteristically focused on fundamentals rather than flashy techniques.

"If I could just do three things that would change your life forever, this is how I would do it," he begins.

The first, predictably, is crawling – the cornerstone of his approach. The second is rocking on hands and knees, a movement that looks deceptively simple, but activates profound connections throughout the body.

"The reason that I would do this," Tim explains as he demonstrates the quadruped rocking movement, "is because this is where strength is built reflexively on the ground. And when we rock back and forth here, we're doing so many wonderful things for the body."

The subtle, rhythmic movement creates system-wide integration: "We're activating the vestibular system through motion. But we're also telling the body where all the joints are and how they're all designed to move together as one whole body."

(The vestibular system is basically your body's built-in balance and spatial awareness tool. Think of it as the tiny gymnasium inside your inner ear! It's made up of fluid-filled loops and chambers that work like a human-sized level tool. When you move your head, this fluid shifts around, telling your brain which way is up and how you're moving through space. This nifty system is why you can close your eyes and still touch your nose, or know if you're upside down on a roller coaster. It's also the reason you feel dizzy after spinning in circles - that fluid keeps sloshing around even after you stop! When your vestibular system works well, you hardly notice it. But when it's off, you might feel dizzy, unsteady, or like the room is spinning. It works together with your eyes and body sensors to keep you balanced and coordinated throughout the day.) - the author

Tim uses an orchestral metaphor to convey the importance of this coordination: "This actually is like putting all the instruments in a symphony together. Every major joint is learning how to play together and move together rhythmically, fluidly. So that there is no one ankle. There is a body that has two ankles, two knees, two hips, two shoulders, a rib cage, and a spine. And they all know how to dance and play together."

As we discuss the movement, Tim notices my attention to foot position during the rocking pattern. This leads to an important observation about toe mobility – a seemingly minor detail with major implications.

"A lot of guys I've trained and I see, can't actually bend their toes," I note, removing my shoes to demonstrate the importance of toe flexibility.

Tim emphasises the significance of this often-overlooked aspect of movement: "All your moving joints are designed to move for a reason. Because they're designed to move. And that allows for an efficient movement of the body."

When joint mobility is lost, compensations cascade throughout the system: "If you lose the ability to move a joint that is designed to move, that means other joints in your body have to make up for the loss of that movement. Which means they are now going to start to work in a way that they weren't intended to."

This compensation pattern has particularly significant consequences in the feet: "The forces that your body generates, which start at the foot, because we walk on our feet, those forces do not travel efficiently through your body like they should if the joints don't move."

The connection between toe mobility and whole-body function exemplifies Tim's integrated view of movement: "If your toes move well, your knees move well, your hips move well, your shoulders move well. Maybe your jaw doesn't hurt. It's crazy, I know, but good moving toes make a good moving body."

For his third foundational movement, Tim introduces what he calls "up and over" – a transitional movement pattern that begins on the back, moves through standing, and ends on the belly, then reverses the sequence.

"The more creative I am on how I want to do this, whether I want to do it like Spiderman, or however I want to do it, the more you do it, the more gaps you fill in in your strength. And you become stronger and stronger and stronger."

The beauty of this movement lies in its adaptability and accessibility: "All it takes is a little bit of time, a little bit of space... If you're creative, you can tie everything together. 10 minutes of that, have a great day. You're going to feel good. You're going to move amazingly. And you'll be strong."

The Mindset Matters Most

Beyond the specific techniques, what stands out in my conversation with Tim is his emphasis on mindset as the ultimate determinant of physical transformation.

When I ask about his advice for overcoming common obstacles to fitness, Tim's answer goes beyond the physical: "The biggest challenge I think for people is that you gotta let go of what you think you know, and be open to a different possibility because I guarantee you everything you want, is inside of you, and it's within your grasp."

This perspective challenges the common belief that solutions lie in external systems or techniques: "It's not outside of you. Like, there is no magic set and reps game. There is no magic exercise. There is no magic diet."

Tim suggests that our beliefs about what's possible largely determine our physical experience: "If you believe that the answer is somewhere else, you'll never find it, and you'll be absolutely right, though, that yeah, you can't do that. You think that your best days are behind you because you're not thinking right."

This message is particularly relevant for men in midlife who may have accepted limitations as inevitable: "Nobody's best days are behind them, unless you've decided that they are. That's because where the brain goes, where the mind goes, the body's going to follow it and do absolutely what you tell it to do."

Tim's approach to fitness isn't just about restoring movement patterns – it's about restoring belief in one's physical potential. By reconnecting with the movement intelligence we all possessed as children, he suggests we can rediscover capabilities we thought were lost to time.

"Your body's a good pet," he says with a smile. "It's like your best friend dog. It'll do what you want it to do, what you tell it to do, and what you enable it to do."

With his Original Strength system, Tim Anderson offers us a training methodology and a philosophy of physical potential – one that starts not with complex exercises or grueling workouts but with the simple movement patterns we all mastered before we could speak. In doing so, he provides a pathway back to the natural strength and mobility that resides within each of us, waiting to be reawakened.

Reflection questions

1. How might focusing on fundamental movement patterns from childhood (breathing, head control, rolling, rocking, and crawling) rather than complex exercise routines change your approach to fitness and overall well-being?

2. Tim Anderson mentions that many men in their forties fall into "the memory trap" of trying to exercise as they did when they were teenagers. In what ways might you be holding onto past fitness approaches that no longer serve your current body and life circumstances?

3. Tim Anderson emphasises the importance of measuring progress through work capacity rather than just weight lifted or reps completed. How might tracking your movement quality and efficiency (like his crawling time measurement) provide more meaningful feedback about your physical development than traditional fitness metrics?

THE IRON TAMER: BENDING STEEL AND SHAPING REALITY

"Nothing and no one can prevent you from improving your self image."
- **Dave Whitley the "Iron Tamer"**

The air in Nashville crackled with a different kind of energy. It wasn't just the crisp Tennessee autumn morning, though that was certainly a factor. It was the anticipation of meeting Dave Whitley, 'The Iron Tamer.' 'I'd first crossed paths with Dave back in 2011, a lifetime ago, at a kettlebell course in South Korea. He was a patient, insightful teacher, laying the foundation for my own kettlebell journey. Now, years later, we were meeting again, this time on the outskirts of Nashville, to delve into the mind of a man who seemed to bend not just steel, but the very fabric of perceived limitations.

Dave Whitley is a man of many facets: author, speaker, performing strongman, and a mentor who guides others to unlock their hidden potential. But beneath these titles lies a core truth: Dave is a master of mindset. He understands that true strength isn't just about physical prowess; it's about the power of the mind to shape reality. As we settled into our conversation, I was eager to uncover the secrets behind his extraordinary achievements and learn how his unique perspective could empower men over 40 to live fortified lives.

'Welcome to Tennessee,' Dave greeted me, his voice warm and inviting. 'I hope you're having a fantastic time here. 'And indeed, we were! 'You've come at the best time of year, 'he added.

Beyond the pleasantries, I sensed a deep well of wisdom, a lifetime of lessons forged in the fires of both physical and mental discipline. I knew this conversation would be more than just an interview; it would be a masterclass in living a life of intention and strength.

'Dave, 'I began, 'you've written books, you're a speaker, you perform incredible feats of strength. How do you fit all these seemingly disparate pieces into your life? 'His answer, as I would soon discover, was a testament to the power of vision, planning, and a fundamental shift in how we perceive life's challenges and opportunities.

The Hulk, Gamma Radiation, and the Spark of Possibility

Dave's fascination with strength wasn't a late-blooming interest; it was a childhood obsession, sparked by the iconic image of Lou Ferrigno as the Incredible Hulk. 'I became fascinated with strength when I was a little kid,' Dave recalled, a hint of nostalgia in his voice. 'Wanted to be the Hulk after seeing Lou Ferrigno on television…'

For a young Dave, the Hulk wasn't just a comic book fantasy; he was a tangible possibility. 'It went from being this comic book fantasy cartoon thing into, I know that's a guy and it's an actor and he's wearing makeup, but that's his real body. And something triggered in my mind that it was possible for a person to be big and strong like the Hulk.'

This realisation sent him on a quest, a quest that revealed the innocent, yet determined, nature of a child's unwavering belief. 'I took the Sunday paper out, and I spread it out, and I'm looking through, and my mum comes in, knowing that this is my regular thing on Sunday, she says, "What are you doing?" Because I didn't have the comics this time, I had the classified section, which, in the internet age, is a lot like Craigslist now, or Facebook Marketplace. So I spread out the classified, and she says, "What are you doing?" I said, "I'm looking for gamma radiation."'

The room filled with a shared chuckle. 'Because I thought that's how you get that way, right? Because that's what I knew from the comics. And in an era before Google, it was very difficult to find gamma radiation. I couldn't even find so much as a radioactive spider in there, right?'

Though his search for gamma radiation proved fruitless, the spark had been ignited. It was the first step in a lifelong pursuit of understanding and mastering human potential. 'I just let it go for a while,' Dave continued, 'And then not too long after that, I saw Ferrigno on television again in a replay of Pumping Iron. And he was there with Franco Colombo and Arnold Schwarzenegger. And so there were these massive guys, and they were doing the training segments. And I realised then that, okay, the way to get big and strong and the way to be able to lift heavy things is to lift heavy things. And that makes you bigger and strong.'

That Christmas, Dave received a set of weights, a tangible symbol of his newfound understanding. 'That started me on the track and that's been 40 plus years ago now,' he said. This simple act, born from a child's innocent dream, laid the groundwork for a life dedicated to strength, both physical and mental. It was the beginning of a journey that would lead him to become the Iron Tamer, a man who not only bent steel but also shaped his own reality.

The Entrepreneurial Strongman: Balancing Passions and Priorities

Dave's journey didn't stop at physical strength; it expanded into a multifaceted career, blending his passions into a sustainable lifestyle. 'Now it's my full-time way of earning a living as an entrepreneur,' Dave explained, 'most entrepreneurs, the successful ones, anyway, will have multiple things that they're involved in that are generating income.'

He's not just a strongman; he's a strategic entrepreneur. 'I wrote a couple of books, like you said, I train people online. I do workshops. I do public speaking and strongman performances as part of a motivational speech. All that stuff combined puts me in a position that I'm able to do what I love to do, what I'm supposed to be doing, what I really feel compelled to do.'

But amidst the diverse roles and income streams, one priority stood above the rest: family. 'It also allows me to spend the majority of my time at home with my son, who will be a year old next week. My wife's also self-employed, so we get to stay home with him.'

This dedication to family led to a significant shift in his career. 'I did own a gym for quite a while. And then a little over a year ago, right before he was born, I got out of the gym business. My lease was up. I said, I don't want to do this thing where I'm leaving the house and being gone for hours at a time. So I set myself up so that I could be at home with him.'

Dave's ability to structure his life around his priorities wasn't a matter of chance; it was the result of meticulous planning. 'Scheduling everything and planning out the week is something that I do every week on Sunday. I sit down with my wife and say, okay, what do we have coming up this week and we plan it out.'

This proactive approach allowed him to manage his diverse responsibilities effectively. 'Being able to fit everything in is a matter of deciding what it is that you want to do, prioritising it, and then planning the time in advance so that you can take incremental steps towards it.'

He emphasised the importance of focused effort, avoiding the pitfalls of multitasking. 'If I'm working on writing the book, it works better for me to say I'm going to allot three hours a week to work on this particular project and this is when that time is happening and I'm not doing anything else but that. So I'm not trying to change a diaper and work on a book at the same time because that's half doing two things.'

Dave's life was a testament to the power of intention and strategic planning, a model for men over 40 seeking to balance their passions and responsibilities. 'So it all comes down really to being a matter of focusing on what's the priority at the moment, 'he concluded. 'And that's how you make it all work.'

The Mindset Shift: From Challenges to Puzzles

Our conversation naturally flowed from the practicalities of scheduling to the deeper realms of perception. I had observed that Dave didn't just manage his time effectively; he managed his mind. And it was this mental agility, this ability to reframe obstacles, that truly set him apart.

'You were talking about planning and focusing, 'I remarked, 'and this wasn't going to be my next question, but it's really important. I'm going to change the order. Because planning and focusing is also very important when someone wants to get healthier and fitter and stronger. I see a lot of guys fail to reach their goals. Because for one, they don't have a specific goal. So if you don't have a goal, you don't know when you reach it. And the other thing, they don't have a plan either. What's your advice to the audience about approaching the matter of getting fitter and stronger over 40 and necessary steps in order to be successful at achieving those goals?'

Dave's response wasn't a typical fitness guru's pep talk. Instead, he offered a profound insight into the power of language and perception. "When you asked me that, my first thought was of many years ago, when I began learning how our words shape our perception of the world around us."

He shared a pivotal moment of realisation. 'And I noticed that a lot of people that were very into seeing the positive in any situation and gleaning the good from it, they wouldn't say the word problem, they would say challenge. And I'm like, that makes sense because problem has this negative connotation or whatever. And I didn't really think that much about it. Until one day, it hit me that a challenge is something that must be overcome. There's a certain level of effort and almost combativeness in it. Either the challenge is going to defeat me or I'm going to defeat the challenge.'

This subtle shift in terminology had a profound impact on Dave's approach to life. 'And in a concentrated attempt to make everything easier in my life, I thought what's a problem then? If that's a challenge, what's a problem? And it took me back to math class. A problem is something that has a solution. And every problem really has multiple solutions. So rather than fight this thing and try to overcome it, what if I just look at it from the standpoint of what's the easiest way to solve this thing that's in front of me?'

He emphasised the transformative power of this linguistic shift. 'And it sounds like semantics, but it's not. On a deeper level that sort of defies words, those are two different feeling mental states, emotional states. And the emotional state that we take on becomes what our experience is.'

Dave then referenced the work of Neville Goddard, a figure who had significantly influenced his understanding of the mind. 'One of the guys that I'm a huge fan of and have studied everything that he's ever written or spoken is a guy named Neville Goddard. And the quote that's coming to mind right now, the quote from Neville is that the words that we speak, and I'm paraphrasing this, the words that we speak and the thoughts that we have and the things that we imagine don't fade into the past. They advance into the future to confront us, right? And so whatever I speak now, whatever I imagine now, whatever I think now, I will encounter later.'

He then explained his evolution from the word problem to the word puzzle. 'So, I don't think of challenges and obstacles that way. I think of them as puzzles to be solved. And I've actually recently shifted from the word problem to the word puzzle. Because a puzzle has a fun connotation to it, right?'

This reframing wasn't just a clever linguistic trick but a fundamental shift in perception, transforming life's obstacles into engaging opportunities for growth. For Dave, life wasn't a battle to be won; it was a series of puzzles to be enjoyed.

The Power of Visualisation: Bending the Red Nail

Dave wasn't just theorising about the power of the mind; he was living it. And he had a particularly striking example to share. 'If you really want to accomplish it, 'he advised, 'I recommend that you get into a relaxed state, close your eyes and really construct a scene of what the end looks like, smells like, feels and if you can give that scene like the tones of reality, then you plant that into your subconscious mind, and it takes a lot of the effort out of it.'

He acknowledged that this might sound unconventional. 'It sounds like some kind of woo, far-out stuff, but I've seen it work time and time again. I've never seen it fail when it's been applied appropriately.'

To illustrate this, he recounted his experience with a specific physical goal: bending the Red Nail.

'And the first place that I really experienced this for myself was in 2013, when I was working on a specific physical goal, ' Dave explained. 'Iron Mind is a company that produces high-quality strength training equipment for those unfamiliar. They offer a series of progressively challenging steel bars, called nails, culminating in the Red Nail. This particular nail is a 5/16-inch (8mm) diameter, seven-inch length of cold-rolled steel. To officially bend the Red Nail, and have your name added to the prestigious list, you must accomplish it under specific conditions: within one minute, using Iron Mind's approved equipment, and with minimal hand wrapping for protection.'

Dave's goal was clear, and he approached it with a blend of physical training and mental rehearsal. 'When I decided that was the thing that I wanted to do, I was also reading a book that Marty Gallagher recommended. It's called Clearing the Path to Victory, and it's about constructing the scene and visualising for athletes. So I started practicing that, and I got so involved in it from a meditative visualisation, being in the imaginal act standpoint, that two different times, not just once, but twice, I shocked myself out of that relaxed trance-like state because I started sneezing from imaginary chalk dust that was in the air from me prepping the nail.'

He painted a vivid picture of his visualisation process. 'So I would go through this whole thing where I was wrapping the nail up and put chalk on my hands. The last thing I would do before I pick it up and bend it in this imaginary act is I'd put the chalk on my hands, I'd rub them together, and I'd clap, and this cloud of dust would come up. I'd pick up the nail and go from there. And that dust cloud in my imagination triggered physical sneezes from me on two different occasions. And it was at that point that I'm like, okay, this has already happened in my mind. It's not even, it's gonna happen. It's already happened.'

The power of his mental imagery was undeniable. 'And in the scene that I had constructed, I was in a room with a group of people. I didn't really see their faces, but there were probably 15 people sitting around in a semi-circle in chairs. And I was bending this thing, and I bent it in less than 30 seconds. I just remember that as long as I come in under 30 seconds, I have plenty of time to play with.'

The reality mirrored his visualisation with uncanny precision. 'You can see the video of the Red Nail bend on my YouTube channel,' Dave stated. 'The scene unfolded exactly as I'd imagined. We were conducting an Old Time Strongman

University workshop, led by my mentor, Grandmaster Strongman Dennis Rogers, and me. Around twenty people were present, arranged in a semi-circle, just as I'd visualised. After bending the nail, an official referee, as appointed by Iron Mind, confirmed the feat. He announced, '17 seconds. 'That was my fastest time ever. The speed was the only deviation from my mental rehearsal; the actual bend was even quicker.'

Dave's story wasn't just a personal anecdote; it was a testament to the power of visualisation, a technique backed by scientific studies. 'And then there was that study that I don't know who did, but they had the three different groups that were shooting basketballs, like this, right? One actually practiced, one mentally rehearsed, and the control group did nothing. And the level of improvement was almost identical between the physical practice and the imaginal practice group. Okay, so if this works for this, what else will it work for?'

He had unlocked a powerful tool, a way to shape his reality through the power of his mind.

Intelligent Training: Adaptation Over Force

Dave's approach to training wasn't about brute force or pushing past perceived limitations; it was about understanding the body's natural capacity for adaptation. 'People associate it with lions, right? The king of beasts,' he explained. 'But what does a lion actually do? They sleep a lot. And when they do hunt, they're efficient. They don't waste energy chasing the strongest prey. They target the easiest catch.' He paused, adding with a touch of humor, 'I was corrected on this, by the way. The lionesses often do the hunting, while the males conserve energy. Which, honestly, is even smarter.'

Dave applied this principle directly to strength training. 'If I want to get stronger,' Dave emphasised, 'I don't need to constantly push against my absolute limits. Imagine your maximum potential as a circle. Sitting on the couch watching Netflix is inside that circle, requiring minimal effort. Moving beyond the circle? That's where injury occurs. So, where does true progress lie? Not lounging on the couch, but also not flirting with the edge of that circle, where breakage happens...'

Dave's approach was about finding the sweet spot, the zone where consistent effort led to sustainable progress. '...and for me, like when I see people talking about kettlebell training specifically and they post pictures of ripped up hands, I'm like, you are bragging about an injury you sustained. That's dumb. Why didn't you stop before you ripped your hands up? Because I'm pushing past my limit. Okay, good for you. What you're doing is losing training time when you do that. You are being so driven by the desire to do something that you are leaving your true desire, which is to attain something, on the table. And that sounds like semantics, but it's not.'

He concluded with a powerful statement about the body's inherent ability to adapt. 'You cannot force your body to adapt to anything. Nor can you prevent it from adapting to whatever activities you participate in.'

The Greatest Achievements: Fatherhood and Impact

As we were nearing the end of our talk, I wanted to understand what truly mattered most to Dave, what he considered his greatest triumphs. 'Let's talk about your three greatest achievements in your life, 'I asked, 'If you can name three.'

He paused, a moment of genuine reflection. 'I'm blindsided by this, ' he admitted, 'Didn't know this was going to be one of the questions.'

'That's good, 'I replied, 'I've managed to surprise you.'

'Number one, greatest achievement for me, 'Dave began, his voice softening, 'and this is going to sound hokey, but I don't care because it's true. Number one, my greatest achievement is having my son be born.'

The depth of his emotion was palpable. 'At the point in my life that he was born, I'll be 50 in November. He will turn one a month before I turn 50. It's our only child. We went through a lot of hardship and difficulty to be able to have him. That's a story for another time.'

He shared how becoming a father later in life had profoundly changed his perspective. 'If I had become a parent in my mid-twenties, I don't think I would have an appreciation for the passage of time as a general factor in my life that I have now. I don't think I would have had an appreciation for him as a human that I do now, because just the wisdom and the experience you achieve as you pay attention to things that happen over the years becomes a part of you.'

Dave's focus wasn't just on his own joy; it was on the legacy he was creating. 'And so now I'm able to look at him and I'm able to look at patterns that I have carried with me through much of my life that didn't serve me, that I've gone in and reprogrammed in my mind. And I'm like, what if we start from a standpoint of never introducing those patterns into his mind and only introducing things into his mind that we believe are going to be beneficial to him? What's he going to be like when he's 20?'

He envisioned a life shaped by positive influences. 'And what kind of story is he going to have to tell just from being exposed to my friends and people that I know? Because I know a huge number of extraordinary people who have had a massive influence on my life. You've talked to several of them on your trip here. And what will it be like when my son's 10 years old and picks up a deck of cards and rips it in half? It's just something that daddy does. Yep. Versus daddy gets up and goes and does whatever a normal thing is.'

'He emphasised that his desire was not to put down anyone, but to create a positive environment for his son. 'This isn't meant as criticism of anyone whose life is different,' he explained, 'but I see it as an opportunity to avoid passing on patterns that didn't serve me well. I believe this realisation—

and including him in this journey—is probably my greatest accomplishment.'

'What are numbers two and three?' I asked.

'I don't know,' he replied, a moment of genuine humility. 'You don't have to rank them,' I reassured him.

'It's, yeah, what's the next one? I forget,' he chuckled. 'But it's closely related,' he continued. 'It's having the opportunity to share ideas, like we're doing now, that might resonate with someone I'll never meet. To inspire them to re-evaluate their own lives and say, "This doesn't serve me anymore. I'm going to change it."'

'Very often,' Dave continued, 'when people get into the 40-ish age bracket, we start thinking that my best years are behind me and this is how my life is and I've just got to ride this thing out until I'm going to keep delaying expressing who I am. I'm going to keep delaying my happiness. And then you wake up one day and you're 70 and never did what you wanted to do. And I don't want to be that guy. Fortunately, my desire not to be that guy has put me in a position where I get to help a whole lot of other people. Even if it's just in some small way.'

He shared a few examples of how he'd positively impacted others. 'Just last week, after a high school show, a young student approached me, asking for a souvenir,' Dave recounted. 'I'd already packed everything away, but I found an extra nail in my bag and gave it to him. His appreciation was genuine, and those moments are incredibly rewarding.'

Dave's second achievement focuses on his ability to positively impact others: "I'm grateful to be in a position where I can have conversations like we're having now that reach people I may never meet in person. When someone hears or reads something I've shared, and it resonates with them enough to change an aspect of their life that isn't serving them—that's deeply meaningful to me."

Then, Dave shared a particularly poignant story. 'Several years ago, I performed at a convention – a sort of comic-con type event, 'he began. 'It was a crowd filled with cosplayers and gamers, and there's a common stereotype that those folks aren't physically active. I didn't find that to be true, but the perception persists. After the show, many people came up to express their appreciation. But one young woman, probably in her early twenties, stood out. She was withdrawn, her posture suggesting a deep unease. Yet, she waited patiently until everyone else had left. When she finally approached, she began to speak…'

'She was talking to me, 'Dave continued, 'and she said, "I've been dealing with depression for a long time. I've been struggling. And I saw you do this show, and it made me realise that I'm not broken. That I can still do things. That I can still be strong. And I just wanted to thank you."'

Dave paused, his voice filled with emotion. 'That was it, 'he said. 'That was the whole exchange. But it meant the world to me. Because that's why I do what I do. It's not about bending steel. It's about bending perceptions, breaking down barriers, and showing people that they're capable of more than they think.'

He added, 'And that's the kind of thing that makes everything else worthwhile. I'm not saying that every show is going to have that kind of impact, but that kind of interaction is what I'm striving for.'

Superhuman Potential

Our conversation concludes with the story behind Dave's book, "Superhuman You," which began as scattered notes and ideas about the connection between mental practices and physical strength.

The project gained momentum after a pivotal interaction with personal development author Joe Vitale, known from the film "The Secret." "Joe sends me a Facebook message," Dave recalls, "and I'm like, 'Okay, somebody's pretending to be Joe Vitale.'"

After confirming it was indeed the real Joe Vitale, they began corresponding, eventually leading to in-person meetings where Dave taught Joe about feats of strength while Joe shared insights on mindset.

During one of these exchanges, Joe asked if Dave had considered writing another book. When Dave mentioned his ideas about connecting strongman principles with concepts from Napoleon Hill, Joe Vitale, and Neville Goddard, Joe responded enthusiastically: "I think that sounds like a great idea for a book... When are you going to send me the rough draft?"

Without fully considering the implications, Dave committed to a mid-February deadline. "He reaches out to shake my hand. And he says, 'I look forward to it.' And I realised as I shook his hand, I just agreed to write a book."

What followed was a creative process that transformed scattered notes into a structured manuscript through an unexpected route – a webinar that became a transcription that became a book. "Within a week, I had this rough draft that I sent to Joe Vitale about a week early," Dave says. "By March 15th, I had a physical copy of it in my hand."

Now, Dave is expanding the book's concepts into a coaching program centered on helping people discover their own unique "superhuman" abilities. "Superhuman – we throw that around. We think Marvel, DC, Star Wars, or any of that stuff," he explains. "But if we look at what superhuman power is in the context of the world that we live in, 'super' means over, above, exhibiting characteristics to an excessive degree; 'human,' we don't need an explanation for, that's us; and 'power' is the ability or capacity to do something."

This definition reveals Dave's ultimate mission – helping others recognise and develop their innate potential: "I'm looking for people who want to take these abilities or the capacity to do something that they have as a human, and elevate that to an extreme or excessive degree, which is what 'super' means, right? I want it to be over, above and beyond what even they thought was possible."

As our formal conversation ends, Dave prepares to demonstrate some of his signature feats of strength – physical manifestations of the mental principles he has shared. But what lingers most powerfully is not the image of bent steel or torn decks of cards, but the integrated philosophy that underlies them – a philosophy that suggests our greatest strength isn't in our muscles but in the focused, directed power of our minds.

Reflection Questions

1. The Language of Possibility: Dave Whitley transformed his perception of obstacles by reframing "problems" as "puzzles" to be solved rather than challenges to be overcome. How might changing your language around difficulties shift your emotional state and approach to fitness goals, career obstacles, or personal challenges you're currently facing?

2. Visualisation as Practice: Dave's story about bending the Red Nail demonstrates how vivid mental rehearsal can powerfully shape physical outcomes. What specific goal in your life could benefit from dedicated visualisation practice, and how might you construct a scene with sensory details that plants this vision in your subconscious mind?

3. Legacy and Impact: At the age of 50, Dave considers his input on his son's development and his ability to positively influence others as his greatest achievements. How has your perception of achievement evolved with age, and what legacy do you want to create in this season of life that transcends conventional measures of success?

STRENGTH BEYOND AGE: THE JOHN BROOKFIELD PHILOSOPHY

> *"I tell my mind, 'This is what I'm going to do.' I don't know how hard or easy it's going to be, but here's the workout of the day."*
>
> **- John Brookfield**

On a beautiful Sunday afternoon in Pinehurst, North Carolina, I am sitting in the home of John Brookfield, strongman, inventor of innovative training systems, and at 60 years of age, living proof that physical capability can improve with time.

"I'm 60 years old now," John tells me with a humble smile, "and I feel blessed. I can do some things now at 60 that I couldn't do when I was 20—just from good training and learning how to stay on task and be a little smarter as I get older."

The Real Deal: John Brookfield's Journey from Showman to Strength Master

You've probably seen the ropes. Those thick, heavy battle ropes that appear in every gym commercial swing back and forth as some athlete gets after it. You might not know that those ropes trace back to one man's genius for understanding how the human body works under stress.

John Brookfield didn't set out to revolutionise fitness. He started as a guy fascinated by what the human body could endure and accomplish. Over the decades, this curiosity transformed him into one of the most respected names in strength and conditioning—a coach whose methods now shape how elite athletes, military units, and weekend warriors approach their training.

Television producers caught on early. Shows like *Good Morning America* and *The Today Show* featured John not just for entertainment, but because viewers could sense something authentic about his approach. Here was a man who understood strength from the inside out.

While his Battle Ropes system gained worldwide recognition—becoming the training tool you see everywhere from CrossFit boxes to NFL facilities—John's true innovation lies in his comprehensive approach to human performance. His Chain Reaction Program, Beyond Bodyweight training, and Brookfield's Barrel training all share a common thread: they prepare you for real-world demands, not just gym numbers.

The military gets this. So do professional sports teams. That's why John regularly works with NFL squads and Special Forces units—groups that can't afford training methods that look impressive but fail under pressure.

In his fifty's John proved that his methods work long-term. Partnering with Kirk Nobles, he pulled a 40,000-pound semi-truck for a full mile in just under 51 minutes—without ropes, using only their bodies and technique. The final quarter-mile was uphill. Think about that the next time someone tells you that real strength peaks in your twenties.

What strikes you most about John isn't his records or TV appearances, though. It's his demeanor. In an industry full of ego and bluster, he remains genuinely approachable—the kind of coach who makes complex concepts feel simple and intimidating challenges feel achievable. His regular appearances at Perform Better summits draw crowds not just for the knowledge, but for the calm confidence he brings to everything he teaches.

This is what real expertise looks like: decades of testing, refining, and proving methods that actually work when it matters most.

The Journey Begins: A kid inspired by an 80-year-old

John's path to strength began with an unlikely inspiration. Though his father was an old-time professional basketball player, it was an elderly gentleman at a local hardware store who sparked John's interest in strength training.

"When I was 16 years old, back in Greenfield, Indiana, there was a gentleman, probably about 80-82 years old, who worked at a hardware store," John recalls. "Even at that age, he could bend 60-penny nails with his hands and drive nails through wood with his bare hands. I remember seeing him in the lumber yard doing that while I was playing high school football, and I thought how cool it was."

Inspired, the young Brookfield got some nails and started trying to bend them himself. Despite having relatively small hands, he developed a goal to cultivate the strongest grip in the world. This focus on grip strength became the foundation of his journey.

Building a Legacy Through Knowledge

John's passion for grip strength led him to author several influential books on the subject. "There's Mastery of Hand Strength, the Grip Master's Manual... I wrote four or five books on grip strength," he explains. These works, still sold by Iron Mind Enterprises, have become foundational texts for grip strength enthusiasts.

His knowledge expanded beyond just grip training. "I wrote a small book on Chinese exercise balls and another comprehensive book on cable pulling with the old strands or cables," he adds. These publications cemented his reputation as not just a performer of strength feats but also as an educator.

The Philosophy of Sustainable Strength

What sets John's approach apart is his emphasis on sustainability and work capacity rather than maximum effort. "I've never tried to push myself to the maximum," he reveals. "I've never tried to pull the heaviest deadlift I could pull. I've never trained to failure, ever."

"I did a drill where I took 220 pounds (100 kilos) and did 12 repetitions every minute for three hours on the leg extension bench. Then I did the same with seated rows—220 pounds, 12 repetitions every minute for three hours."

His card-tearing records remain unbroken: "I tore through 100 decks of cards in two minutes and 15 seconds for the Today Show. And at a festival, I tore through 61 decks in 60 seconds." For perspective, he notes that the average construction worker might struggle to tear through just 20 cards, especially considering modern cards are plastic-coated, not paper like in the old days.

Among his metal-bending feats, John bent 520 sixty-penny nails (each about the size of a pencil) into U-shapes in about an hour and a half at the Glasgow, Kentucky Highland Games. He's also created artistic sculptures, including "Samson's Harp"—a 20-foot stick of steel from a tractor-trailer that he rolled into a huge heart.

Priorities Beyond Strength

Despite his strength accomplishments, John's priorities remain clear when asked about his three greatest achievements:

"The first one is my faith since I was about 21 years old, and I've done full-time ministry. That was by far the greatest achievement," he says without hesitation.

"Then I'd have to say being married to my wife, Sherry, for 31 years. And then probably when my daughter was born 23 years ago."

His strong faith and family foundation have provided the support system for his 44-year strength journey.

Wisdom for the Over-40 Athlete

What advice does John offer to those over 40 who want to get back into training? His first suggestion might surprise you.

"Start with your feet—get into a kind of barefoot lifestyle," he recommends. "If you look at a strong and healthy foot, you see that the toes and the heel are at the same level. It doesn't have arch supports or a jacked-up heel like most shoes today."

He suggests cautiously transitioning to a more natural foot position through minimalist, zero-drop shoes that allow the toes to spread naturally. "One of the foundations of strength and longevity is to start with proper feet," he explains, noting that products like toe spacers can help rehabilitate feet damaged by years of wearing improper footwear.

Once the feet are addressed, John advises finding physical activities you enjoy: "I tell people to do something they like. If you enjoy being outside, running or cycling is great. But I prefer combining cardiovascular work with strength—things like rope work and kettlebells that use your whole body while still providing cardiovascular benefits."

The Work Capacity Concept

Central to John's training philosophy is the concept of work capacity—an approach that values sustained effort over short bursts of intensity.

"Let's say you go to a construction site with migrant farm workers. They're not athletes. They've never done a bench press or run a marathon. But they're in the hot sun for 10-12 hours. Take many good athletes or fitness people, put them out there with those workers, and they won't last a tenth of the time."

John believes in combining proper physical training with "good old work, " which farmers or roofers do daily. He encourages setting the mind like a GPS with a predetermined destination, regardless of conditions.

"I tell my mind, 'This is what I'm going to do.' I don't know how hard or easy it's going to be, but here's the workout of the day—just like the farm worker who knows he'll be in the field from 7 AM until 6 PM."

He contrasts this with popular circuit training: "I like circuits, rounds, and intervals because they burn fat and provide good scientific training. But the drawback is that as you perform each exercise for 40 seconds, you switch to something else before it gets really hard. You're letting yourself off the hook each time before things get difficult."

"Real life doesn't work that way," John emphasises. "Real life presses into you and doesn't quit. You have to build up, relax, and sustain."

Perhaps most importantly, John stresses the value of staying calm under pressure—a skill developed through practice and mental preparation.

"You teach yourself how to relax," he says. "A lot of that comes from knowing how long you'll be in a difficult situation. When you don't know how long something will last and keep hoping it will end, that's when your mind starts breaking. But if you know you'll be at a tough drill for two hours, you can prepare mentally for the challenge."

As we prepare to head out to John's training area, his philosophy resonates clearly: strength isn't just about maximum effort but about sustainable power, work capacity, and the mental fortitude to stay calm under pressure. At 60, John Brookfield continues to demonstrate that with the right approach, our physical capabilities need not diminish with age—they can actually improve.

A Lesson in Real Strength

Our interview wrapped up, and John gestured toward his garage. "Come on, let me show you some things."

Within minutes, I found myself in a position I'd never experienced—braced in a one-arm push-up position with me feet up on the wall, and my free hand gripping a thick 38mm/1.5 inch rope threaded through John's homemade contraption of PVC pipes mounted on a wooden platform. The setup looked simple enough: pull 20 meters/66 feet of rope through two pipes that create natural resistance as the rope slides around them. Simple in concept. Brutal in execution.

Over a minute later, I finally pulled the last few feet through and dropped to my knees, relieved it was over. That's when I heard John's voice, calm as ever: "Good. Now change arms." Right.

By the time I finished the second round, I understood something fundamental about John's approach to training. This wasn't about isolated muscle groups or impressive lifting numbers. Every fiber of my body had been working overtime—one arm pulling against serious resistance while the other fought to maintain that awkward wall position and resist gravity, my core straining to keep everything aligned, my legs burning as they pushed against smooth concrete with minimal grip. It felt like hanging off a cliff edge, waiting for a rescue that never comes. No relief, no pause, no way to cheat the system. Every time I found a moment's respite, it vanished almost immediately. "Once you can do three rounds per arm without a break between sides," John said, "you'll be in all right shape."

Thanks, John. I thought I was already in decent shape.

The "warm-up" complete, he led me to his battle ropes—30 meters/98 feet of thick rope that meant 15 meters per arm of non-stop movement. John's standard test: two minutes straight. The longest I'd ever managed was one miserable minute. By 90 seconds, the rope barely made waves. At two minutes, I couldn't have defended myself against a determined toddler.

"See," John said with that knowing grin, "being strong and lifting heavy is great, but you want a body that can go the distance too."

Later, as we worked through some kettlebell drills, I couldn't stop wondering how this 60-year-old in baggy shorts and a T-shirt had so thoroughly humbled me. I'd walked in thinking I was reasonably fit and strong. John had shown me another level entirely.

I was grateful for the lesson. Every now and then, we need someone to remind us not to get comfortable with our achievements—to keep pushing toward something better in everything we do.

Reflection Questions

1. How might John's "never training to failure" philosophy challenge your current fitness approach? Consider areas where pursuing sustainable strength rather than maximum effort could benefit your long-term health and performance.

2. John emphasises the importance of "staying calm under pressure" during sustained physical challenges. Think about a time when your mental state affected your physical performance. How could you apply his principles of mental preparation to improve your resilience in challenging situations?

3. The concept of "work capacity" suggests training your body to sustain effort over time rather than excelling at short bursts of intensity. How might you incorporate this principle into your daily routine, even outside formal exercise sessions?

THE MIND-BODY CONNECTION WITH BILL LEE-EMERY

"Everything in life is innocent. Life, death, and everything in between, it's purely an event. But it's what I make of that event that will either spiral me up or spiral me down."
- Bill Lee-Emery

A Journey Through Cancer

When I sat down with Bill Lee Emery in his home, I was struck by the peaceful energy that surrounded him despite the challenging journey he had recently traveled. At 73 years old, Bill had just emerged from a battle with throat cancer—though he would be quick to correct me on my use of the word "battle." With 40 years of experience in mindset coaching, emotional well-being, and working with elite athletes, Bill approached his cancer diagnosis with a unique perspective that would transform what could have been a devastating experience into one of profound growth and learning.

"In July, I was diagnosed with throat cancer," Bill shared, sipping water from the glass he kept constantly by his side—a new habit formed during his treatment. "I've never spent a night in a hospital in my life. I've never had a major illness. So at my age, it was a bit of a shock."

What happened next was what Bill described as "a completely new hero's journey." His doctor highlighted two critical factors that would make a difference in his recovery:

support and mindset. Fortunately, Bill had both. His partner Julie provided unwavering support, and his decades of mindset work gave him tools that would prove invaluable.

Becoming a Servant to the Body

One of Bill's first revelations was the need to become a "servant to his body." This meant listening to what his body needed and responding without resistance.

"If my body needed something, I wouldn't argue with it," he explained. "For example, I don't normally pee during the night. That's never been an issue for me. But during treatment, if my body woke me up at 2:30 and said 'I want to pee,' I wouldn't argue with it. I wouldn't say 'no, I'll wait till morning.' I'd just get up and do it."

This servant mindset extended to his approach to treatment. Though Bill had spent the last 40-50 years embracing what many call "alternative medicine"—acupuncture, naturopathy, homeopathy, meditation—he now had to accept a treatment path that included chemotherapy and radiation. This wasn't easy for someone who rarely even took an aspirin for a headache.

"For this period of time, I am a servant of my body," he emphasised. "I need to give my body the things that it needs, whether I want to do it or not."

The Power of Personal Narrative

A fundamental principle that guided Bill through his experience was his awareness of the narratives he created around his diagnosis and treatment.

"Everything in life, every event in my life, is innocent. It means nothing," Bill explained. "It's what I make of that event that will either spiral me up or spiral me down."

"When first diagnosed, Bill made a pivotal choice: 'I can either view this as a curse or transform it into a blessing. The choice is mine alone. I refused to let it be a curse. Somehow, I was determined to make it a blessing.'"

This choice extended to how he spoke about his cancer with others. "When I tell people I had cancer, some people say 'oh my god, how awful.' I say no, mine is 90 percent curable, it's manageable, and I'm going to deal with it."

Bill was also mindful of the stories others tried to impose on his experience. "I was really careful about other people's stories about cancer, because most people have some story about cancer, whether it's their own or somebody else's. But I wasn't going to let anyone piss in my swimming pool."

Talking to the Body

Perhaps one of the most unique aspects of Bill's approach was his practice of talking directly to his body—something he had been doing for 40 years.

"I would tell my body, 'Okay, body, it's a Wednesday, we're going to get chemo today,'" he explained. "My body knows it, but I want to have a really close connection with my body."

During treatments, he would tell his body to "take the good things that my body needs from the treatment and let go of all the other things as quickly as my immune system, my lymphatic system can take care of."

For those who might find this practice strange, Bill offered this perspective: "If you've got a dog, or a cat, or a pet, or plants, or a partner or a child that you talk to, you have a relationship with them. And a relationship is a two-way thing."

He continued, "I'm going to have my body for my entire life. So in my view, my relationship with my body needs to be as close and as intimate and as trusting and as vulnerable as is possible."

This approach stood in stark contrast to how many approach illness. "Some people, when they have cancer, they'll wage a war against their cancer," Bill noted. "And that is the absolute opposite of my approach."

He explained why: "When you start a war against anything, whether it's against drugs or terrorism or poverty, none of those wars ever come to an end, and both sides ramp up their armaments."

Instead, Bill embraced a profound connection with his body: "I don't have a war against my body, I talk to my body, because it's me and my body going through this. I'm not going to fight it, I want to be good friends with it."

Managing the Experience

The cancer treatment process was grueling: seven weeks of radiation (five days a week) and chemotherapy (once a week). To manage this challenging period, Bill developed several practical strategies.

First, he broke time into manageable chunks: "I'd break the week into seven days. Every day, I broke it into four parts. Morning. Afternoon, evening, and nighttime. And I had to manage each one separately."

This approach allowed him to focus on the immediate challenge rather than becoming overwhelmed by the entire journey. "When I wake up in the morning, I've just got to manage myself until midday. And then lunchtime, I've got to manage myself until dinnertime."

Bill also invited "human angels" into his life—people who showed up with kindness and generosity. From fellow choir members who helped with yard work to healthcare providers who went above and beyond, Bill and Julie found that "once you make an intention about something, people will just show up."

Perhaps most importantly, Bill practiced deep gratitude for even the smallest victories. "My gradient for gratitude just went up," he shared. "Small, little things—every meal was a victory, and every poo was a bonus."

Slaughtering Sacred Cows

One of the most powerful lessons from Bill's journey was his willingness to question long-held beliefs that no longer served him—what he called "slaughtering sacred cows."

For 45 years, Bill had not eaten red meat. "This became part of my identity," he explained. But during chemotherapy, his red blood cells were severely depleted. After consulting with a nutritionist friend who suggested red meat might help raise his protein levels, Bill faced a difficult choice.

"This is maybe a sacred cow I have to slaughter in the service of my body," he realised. "So I decided I was going to start to eat bits of red meat, little bits, and see how my body dealt with that."

This experience taught him an important lesson: "There may be a context where something is really useful and you stick to it, but when we hold that to be an absolute and we don't evaluate whether it's still useful, that absolute can actually be dangerous."

Finding Wonder in Small Details

During the five anxious days between Bill's PET scan and receiving his results, he experienced what he described as "a near-death experience without having a near-death experience."

"Every day I'd look at things, and I'd look at a tree or a leaf or something, and I'd be full of the wonder of a five-year-old," he recalled. "And it was almost like I was stoned or something.

It was just like, 'wow, look at this.' And for a long time, many days, not just those five days, no day was ordinary."

This heightened awareness became a gift that Bill wanted to maintain. "If I looked at a leaf, for example, I would notice the veins, I would notice small things, and when I would do that, it would bring me back to this 'wow,' almost trippy space."

He recognised this as a pathway to ongoing appreciation of life: "If I want to trip out, I've just got to find a plant and just look at the detail, find a cloud, look at the detail of that, and it brings me to this—no day is ordinary."

Three Principles to Live By

As our conversation drew to a close, I asked Bill to share three actionable principles that readers could implement immediately, whether facing health challenges or simply seeking to live more fully.

1. Remember that every event is innocent. "Everything is innocent, every event in our life is innocent. It's the meaning that we place in it that's really going to spiral us up or spiral us down. So take great care about the meaning that you're placing on anything that happens to you."

2. Take charge of your emotional responses. "Our life isn't emotionally flat. It does go up and down. So we have to deal with our anger, fear, sadness, and joy. Rather than saying 'I'm angry,' it's more useful to go, 'How am I expressing my anger?' Because fear is a verb. So is sadness. So is anger."

3. Be the best friend to your body. "Learn to hug your body. Start a really deep, intimate, and beautiful connection with your body. It is yours. So don't fight it, don't have a war against this part or this part. Get to love it. And that can be a process of learning—everything I'm talking about here is a learnable skill. If I've learned it, you can learn it."

The Blessing in Disguise

When I left Bill's home that day, I carried with me a profound sense that I had witnessed something rare: a person who had transformed what many would consider a tragedy into a source of wisdom and growth.

As Bill put it, "I didn't want to waste this experience. I wanted to literally squeeze the lemon and get all the juice out of this. Because if I was going to go through it, I may as well get some really valuable things."

His friend, who had stage four prostate cancer, had said something similar: "It's weird, Bill, but this has been one of the biggest blessings in my life."

Perhaps that's the ultimate lesson from Bill's journey—that our greatest challenges, when approached with the right mindset, can become our greatest teachers.

"Whatever happens in our life," Bill concluded, "it's neither good nor bad. "It's what we make of our circumstances that will either elevate us or send us into a downward spiral." And we got that choice."

Reflection Questions

1. What "sacred cows" might you be holding onto that no longer serve you?

2. How do you currently speak to your body? What might change if you approached it as your closest friend?

3. Think of a challenging situation in your life. What meaning are you attaching to it? Could you choose a different meaning?

4. When did you last take time to notice the small details in your environment? How might regular practice of this awareness enrich your life?

5. How might breaking difficult periods into smaller, manageable chunks help you navigate your own challenges?

THE WAY OF DISCIPLINE: CAMERON QUINN'S MARTIAL ARTS JOURNEY

"It's not the big things that count. It's not the huge events that make the difference. It's the daily consistent effort. Chugging away, little bit at a time." - **Cameron Quinn**

Finding the Path

"I just tagged along," Cameron Quinn says with a smile, recalling the seemingly insignificant decision that would shape the rest of his life. It was 1971 on Australia's Gold Coast, and his mother had taken his four older sisters to learn self-defense at one of only two martial arts schools in the entire region. Rather than stay home alone, the young Cameron decided to come along.

"The funny thing was, they were completely not interested," he laughs. "But I jumped in the back of the class and I started to train and I was hooked straight away."

That small dojo, run by instructor Frank Everett, was where Cameron first encountered Kyokushin Karate – a traditional Japanese martial art known for its rigorous training and full-contact approach. What began as a casual introduction would evolve into a lifelong passion and eventually take him around the world.

The journey wasn't without interruptions. In 1972, Cameron's father was seconded to Europe for work, and

Cameron found himself at St. Peter's College boarding school in Brisbane for two years. During this time, his training became inconsistent – "those two years were almost a blank," he admits candidly.

But when he returned, something had changed. The hunger for training had only grown stronger during his absence. "I was really hungry to start training again," he recalls, his voice brightening at the memory. "I was young, my body was growing, so I was itching to burn up energy."

His instructor, Frank, had expanded to three schools across the Gold Coast – Miami, Labrador, and Southport – creating an opportunity to train somewhere seven days a week. Cameron seized it fully, embarking on a training schedule that would exhaust even seasoned athletes.

The Seven-Day Commitment

Cameron paints a picture of extraordinary dedication when I ask about his early training regimen. "I was training seven days a week," he says matter-of-factly, as though it were the most natural thing in the world.

His parents initially supported this enthusiasm, dropping him off at various dojos scattered across the Gold Coast. But even the most supportive parents have their limits. "In the end, they just said enough's enough. Seven days too much."

Rather than reduce his training, Cameron found another way. "I used to hitchhike," he explains. "Fortunately, most of the drivers who stopped for me were fellow karate practitioners who recognised me from the dojos. The community looked out for its own." He would travel up and down the coast, moving between dojos with nothing but his gi (uniform) and an insatiable desire to learn.

This level of commitment – seven days a week, multiple locations, hitchhiking when necessary – reveals something fundamental about Cameron's approach to martial arts from the very beginning. While others might see rigorous training as a burden, he embraced it fully, turning potential obstacles into another part of the journey.

Journey to the Source

As Cameron progressed in his training, his thoughts turned toward the source. Mas Oyama – the founder of Kyokushin Karate – had become something of a mythical figure to the teenage practitioner. Not just any instructor would do; Cameron wanted to train with the master himself.

"In grade 11, grade 12, I decided I wanted to go to Japan and train with Mas Oyama," he explains. The idea might have seemed far-fetched for a teenager in 1970s Australia. He notes that the Gold Coast was not yet an international destination – "the only tourism on the Gold Coast was from Victoria and Sydney," and cultural exchange with Japan was limited.

With characteristic determination, Cameron began working weekends as a hotel porter, doing room service deliveries to save money for the trip. But the financial reality quickly became apparent: "I worked out it doesn't matter how much I save, I'm not going to be able to go and stay in Japan for very long."

Rather than abandon his dream, Cameron found another approach. "I tried to think about a way that I could go to Japan and have someone else pay me to do it."

The opportunity came through an unexpected connection – a Japanese exchange student named Shuji Ozeki whom Cameron had met. Shuji suggested applying for a Rotary Exchange Scholarship, and Cameron seized the chance. His successful application secured him a year in Japan with accommodation, education, and food covered.

"So during that year," he says with unmistakable satisfaction, "the most important thing was to go and train with Mas Oyama. Every opportunity I had, I would go and train with him."

The Living Legend

When I ask about Mas Oyama, Cameron's voice is reverent. The founder of Kyokushin was more than just a teacher; he was, as Cameron puts it, "a larger than life figure."

"Although there were martial arts schools in America before Mas Oyama went there in the fifties, he was the one who essentially introduced karate in a big way to the world," Cameron explains. "He had schools all over the world, influenced largely by his incredible personality, drive, belief, and power in karate."

Oyama's reputation was built on demonstrations that seemed to defy human capability. So extraordinary were some of his feats that many dismissed them as fabrications or exaggerations. But Cameron, who has spoken with many of Oyama's contemporaries, offers a different perspective:

"Quite often, a lot of people say it's not true, it can't be true. There's plenty of people around who were eyewitnesses... who confirmed that in fact, a lot of these stories, which seemed too incredible to believe, were quite true."

For the 17-year-old Cameron, training directly with such a figure was transformative. It wasn't just about learning techniques but about absorbing a philosophy and approach to martial arts that would influence his entire life.

The Bridge Between Worlds

Cameron's time in Japan became just the first of several extended training periods in the country. He returned in 1979 for four months and again in 1984 for three months as a live-in student of Oyama, immersing himself completely in the practice.

During these stays, his linguistic abilities deepened alongside his martial arts training. "I studied Japanese in Japan when I was there, and also I did my degree in Japanese at the University of Queensland," he explains, highlighting how his passion for the martial art extended to the language and culture that surrounded it.

This dual expertise – in both Kyokushin Karate and the Japanese language – positioned Cameron as a natural bridge between these worlds. When he returned to Australia and began teaching, his students naturally turned to him with questions about terminology and the deeper meanings behind the practice.

"At some stage, my students started to ask me questions," he recalls. "'Can we get a translation of the Japanese words, or what does this mean, or what does that mean?'"

What began as simple handouts about terminology evolved as students asked deeper questions: "Can you explain the meaning of the names of the kata?" The process snowballed from there. "That's where it started. So I thought there's no point in stopping now."

Drawing on the detailed notes he had kept during his training in Japan, Cameron began compiling what would eventually become his book, "The Budo Karate of Mas Oyama." The book goes beyond mere techniques to explore the philosophical underpinnings of the martial art.

"I introduced the connection between the martial arts origins and Indian yoga philosophy," he explains, "because whilst we recognise that many aspects of martial arts come from China, where did China get them? Many aspects of the Chinese martial arts, particularly the internal breathing systems and so on, all came from India."

This perspective reflects Cameron's holistic understanding of martial arts – not just as isolated techniques or traditions, but as part of a broader tapestry of human physical and spiritual development that spans continents and millennia.

Beyond the Dojo: The Habit of Discipline

When our conversation turns to how martial arts has influenced his life beyond the dojo, Cameron's answer is immediate and emphatic: "Discipline."

The word seems to carry special significance for him. "If you do train seriously regularly, then what seems to be very normal for you is actually quite challenging for a lot of people," he observes. "You don't realise that until you step outside the dojo and you see how difficult some people find just to establish a regular training habit, or just to establish certain behavioral habits."

For Cameron, the habits formed through consistent martial arts training – showing up day after day, pushing through discomfort, maintaining focus and commitment – create a foundation that supports excellence in all areas of life.

This emphasis on habit formation echoes throughout our conversation. Just as Dan John speaks of making oneself "a slave to good habits," Cameron sees habitual discipline as the invisible architecture that shapes a life. What seems extraordinary to others – training seven days a week as a teenager, hitchhiking between dojos, traveling to Japan to train with the master – was simply the natural expression of habits he had deliberately cultivated.

The parallels to religious practice are not lost on him. "When I was a little boy, we grew up with Sunday school and church school and going to church," he reflects. The regularity and ritual of martial arts training offers something similar – a structured practice that provides both framework and meaning.

In an age where many seek quick transformations and overnight success, Cameron Quinn's journey offers a different wisdom: the power of showing up consistently, day after day, year after year. The seemingly small habit of attending a single karate class – because he "just tagged along" – set in motion a lifetime of discipline, achievement, and deeper understanding that continues to this day.

The Three-Legged Chair

Cameron's vision of martial arts is holistic and integrated, encompassing multiple dimensions of human experience. "I tend to find that the martial arts, it's three legs on a chair," he says. "You have the physical, the spiritual, and the technical, and they all work together because they all support each other."

The physical component provides a foundation of health and wellness: "More important in life is developing a consistent habit of being healthy and being fit."

Yet Cameron is quick to challenge simplistic equations of health with happiness: "Some people say, if you don't have your health, you have nothing. But I don't believe that. I think health is very important, but I've met too many healthy people who aren't happy to know that there's no connection. Being healthy does not make you happy. It's a good foundation. It's a good start."

The technical aspects of martial arts shape not just fighting ability but one's entire presence in the world: "It allows you to walk straight, stand up with good posture, pull your shoulder blades together. All these serve to make you to give you a presence in society so people don't want to pick on you. And if they do, you have the technique to deal with it."

The third dimension – what might be called spiritual or mental – represents another interesting cultural bridge. "It's interesting. In English we say the mental side or the spiritual side. In Japanese, essentially the word's one. There's no separation. Because the reality of true spiritual training is, it's actually a mental thing. You have to deal with your mental habits and your mental issues."

This integrated approach provides not just physical skills but an entire philosophical framework for living. "We have the dojo kun, which is on the wall, which is the training oath. And if there's seven precepts in that, and if you were to just seriously take those precepts as an instruction for life you have a religion right there."

The result can be transformative, especially for young people: "I get kids walking to the dojo, or their parents bring them in, almost exasperated, 'I don't know what to do.' And within just a couple of weeks, they're going, 'This is magic. What happened?'"

Cameron's answer is straightforward: "By teaching children to earn their achievements in the dojo, rather than giving them everything, we witness powerful and transformative growth."

The Ever-Evolving Practice

At 61, Cameron's relationship with martial arts has evolved, but his commitment hasn't diminished. "I have my little program that I do at home," he explains when I ask about his current training regimen. "Sometimes I do more than other days. It's a simple program which is not super intense, but it's challenging and it lasts for about one hour."

The consistency remains: "On a good day, I'll do that full hour. Sometimes I won't have time. So I just have maybe 15 minutes of exercise. I try to do something every day. And then I'm in the dojo pretty well six days a week."

His reflections on how his approach has changed over the decades reveal a thoughtful adaptation to life's seasons. "I remember back when I first opened my dojo, and the intensity at which we trained was quite amazing. It really was," he recalls with a hint of nostalgia. "I still get people contact me after 30 years and they say, 'You know what, I used to train in those days in the old dojo in Margaret Street or in the hangar dojo in Brisbane... since then, they've traveled all over the world, train with all kinds of people and never once have they found a place that has that intensity.'"

That intensity was something Cameron imported directly from his training in Japan, creating an environment where even seasoned fighters were challenged: "We would get guys coming to the dojo, kickboxers for example, and they had some notion that they were going to show us up. If you wear a gi, they think you're soft. So they'd come into the dojo and, they'd have their wraps on and they'd have their singlet and they're going to tear the dojo apart. And within an hour, they're begging for a rest. They can't even keep up with just what was literally our warm up."

But priorities change with age and experience: "Now, let's go forward. Now that's 35, 40 years ago. Now I don't train anywhere near as much, because the objective then was to get fit, get hard, fight, win tournaments, this sort of thing. Now my objective is, don't get injured."

At 61, his goals have shifted: "Don't get injured, stay flexible, stay healthy, make sure I can sit with a straight spine. And then anything else is a bonus. And if I can do some push-ups and sit-ups and squats and still do my kata. And still train with the guys. And I still love to get on the mat and roll around and wrestle with guys who are 30, 40 years younger. So as long as I can still enjoy all that, that's enough."

This evolution reveals a mature understanding of martial arts as a lifelong journey with different phases: "I think it's good to have competition. In the Kyokushin style of competition there's no padding. It's bare fists, it's knockout, it's full contact. It really is important to develop that courage."

But wisdom includes knowing when to transition: "There's a time and place for that because there's lessons to be learned from that. But there's also a time and place to know when to retire and know when to take your life a little more gently physically and a little more seriously spiritually and psychologically and emotionally."

The One Breath Approach

When I ask what advice he would give to someone over 40 looking to reclaim or establish physical activity in their life, Cameron's answer reflects both his philosophical depth and practical wisdom.

"It depends on the individual," he begins, acknowledging there's no universal formula. "Just like there's no diet is perfect for everyone. There's no spiritual path is perfect for everyone."

He identifies two distinct profiles, each requiring a different approach: "Some people who've come from a very physically active youth, and then they go to uni, they get married, they have a family, they go from one extreme to the other. For them it can be dangerous, because their memory is that 'I used to be a champion athlete,' so now I want to get back into it, and they go back into it a little too hard, too fast."

The second group faces different challenges: "For people who have never been active it's coming the other way."

Cameron offers a beautiful metaphor from the world of art: "Have you ever been to Florence in Italy where Michelangelo's David is? And you know the prisoners? Those stone statues that are incomplete? It's like that. Some sculptors start with a big block of marble and chip away, and others start with a wire frame and they build on, but the finished product is the same. So some people have to learn how to bring it down, some people have to learn to bring it up."

But regardless of starting point, his fundamental advice is strikingly minimalist: "The easiest way, I think, honestly the best way is to just start with a single breath. You're completely sedentary and you want to get started, then set your alarm just five minutes earlier, and you get up and you walk out and you take a single breath."

This seemingly small step contains profound significance: "And if you do that consistently for one week, you've really achieved something amazing because you're beginning to change habits. And it's all about habits."

Cameron understands the depth of entrenched patterns: "For 20 years, it's been digging in and that groove's quite deep. So you're not going to get out of that groove straight away. So what you do is you just start off with a single breath. One thing. Not 10, not 20."

He contrasts this with the common all-or-nothing approach: "Sometimes people just go from Monday, 'I'm doing this and this. I give up alcohol. I give up sugar. I give up bread. I go to the gym five days a week.' And then after two weeks, it slows down. It's just three days now."

Instead, Cameron advocates a progressive timeline: "You got to get over the first four days. If you can be consistent for four days, then your next goal is four weeks. And if you can be consistent for four weeks, then your next goal is four months. And if you can be consistent for four months you've completely changed that groove, that habitual groove."

The path builds gradually from that single breath: "After a few days, single breath, one pushup. After a few more days, a couple of breaths. One pushup, sit down, close your eyes, another breath. And then you just build on just a little bit at a time, chip away, build on."

The Unity of Mind and Body

Perhaps most intriguing is Cameron's insight into the relationship between physical and mental flexibility: "The thing that you see most that makes someone old is the loss of mobility. As people get older, they get stiff. And what starts their stiffness is their mental stiffness."

He directly connects psychological rigidity and physical limitation: "They become opinionated. Take a look at people who become stiff before their time; they're opinionated, very narrow-minded, and have all these crazy, stiff beliefs. So they become very rigid in their minds."

The remedy begins not with physical stretching but mental flexibility: "The first thing you can do is just learn to just let go of things. And just be more relaxed in your mindset, more flexible with your thinking, then all of a sudden your body lets go as well, and the next thing you know, you can regain the youthfulness simply by changing your mindset."

This holistic view of aging and renewal reflects Cameron's integration of Eastern and Western perspectives, of martial arts and broader life philosophy: "It's not the big things that count. It's not the huge events that make the difference. It's the daily consistent effort. Chugging away, little bit at a time, little bit at a time. Fall off the track, doesn't matter, go back to it. Don't beat yourself up, doesn't matter."

His story reminds us that extraordinary lives are often built not on dramatic moments of inspiration but on the steady accumulation of disciplined habits – the daily decisions to train, to learn, to grow that, over time, transform not just the body but the entire person.

Reflection questions

1. How has your understanding of discipline evolved over your lifetime? In what ways might approaching discipline as a daily habit rather than occasional bursts of effort transform your personal growth journey?

2. Cameron describes martial arts as a "three-legged chair" of physical, technical, and spiritual dimensions. How balanced are these three elements in your life pursuits, and which leg might need strengthening to create greater stability and fulfillment?

3. The thing that you see most that makes someone old is the loss of mobility. As people get older, they get stiff. And what starts their stiffness is their mental stiffness." How might cultivating mental flexibility in your beliefs and perspectives directly impact your physical well-being and overall approach to aging?

THE BEAST TAMER: SHAUN CAIRNS ON BUILDING STRENGTH THAT LASTS

> *"Before I learned the art, a punch was just a punch, and a kick, just a kick. After I learned the art, a punch was no longer a punch, a kick, no longer a kick. Now that I understand the art, a punch is just a punch and a kick is just a kick."* -
> **Bruce Lee**

From Rugby Fields to the World Stage

The morning sunshine streams through the window as I sit down with Shaun Cairns in his home in South Africa. At first glance, Shaun's robust build and calm demeanor speak of decades of disciplined physical training, but his approachable warmth immediately puts me at ease.

"Shaun is a StrongFirst certified Master Instructor," I explain to the camera. "He travels the world teaching kettlebell, barbell, and bodyweight strength courses for trainers to get qualified."

Shaun nods with a modest smile. "I've got a family. I've got four kids. All train. Involved in what we do. I've even got my father training. He's in his 70s, and he joins me twice a week, trains with kettlebells, and sometimes uses heavier weights than the young guys do."

This multigenerational approach to strength training – spanning from his children to his septuagenarian father – offers an immediate glimpse into Shaun's philosophy: strength isn't just for the young or athletically gifted; it's a lifelong practice accessible to anyone willing to approach it intelligently.

Born and raised in South Africa, Shaun's journey into strength training began through sports, as it does for many. "In South Africa, we have different sports at school. One of them is rugby – most important – and at school, we played rugby," he explains. "You could only get out of playing rugby if you had a doctor's certificate; otherwise, you played. Sport is an integral part of growing up in South Africa."

From rugby, Shaun branched out into swimming, competing at "a reasonably high level" before gravitating toward weight training in the late 1980s. "When I went to university, I really got into the weight training side of things at that stage. Stopped playing rugby, taking a bit of a break, and started really training with the weights."

His dedication to strength training led to an unexpected venture: "In my final year of university, I actually entered a bodybuilding competition. It's one of the things that few people know about me."

Shaun reflects on this phase with characteristic honesty: "It was a novice competition. It was fun to do. And it's like a lot of things – you don't know if you like it unless you try it. I enjoyed the experience for what it was. Not so much that I'd do it again; it's quite hard on the body. And I came fourth in the men's open novice and had a lot of fun."

After university, Shaun continued weight training while returning to rugby at the club level. The dual focus on both sport and structured strength training would become a pattern throughout his life, combining practical athletic application with systematic strength development.

The Search for Something Different

As our conversation continues, Shaun reveals how a series of life events – including a motorcycle accident in 1997 and starting a family – led him to build a home gym. "With the first child born at the end of '97, we didn't have much time. The time it took to get to the gym and back, you could get a whole training session done at home."

By 2003, Shaun and his wife had four children and had developed their home gym into a space where they could train "before the kids woke up," giving them "a little bit of time to re-energise."

During this period, Shaun began to feel the accumulated effects of his rugby days. "When you're young playing sports, especially a contact sport like rugby, you end up doing things to your body that you only pay for later on. And now, getting into my early thirties, I was starting to pay for some of the things I'd done. And I needed something different."

That "something different" appeared unexpectedly in a South African Men's Health magazine – an article about kettlebells. Intrigued, Shaun ordered a set of kettlebells and instructional materials from "this Russian guy" named Pavel Tsatsouline.

"I didn't know how this was going to change my view of training," Shaun admits.

At this point in his life, Shaun was a successful entrepreneur running two companies in risk management and distribution services. Kettlebell training was just a side interest – something he "played with" for about a year, following along with Pavel's video and asking his wife how his form looked.

The turning point came when a friend – an injured former Springbok rugby player – sought Shaun's advice. Shaun recommended kettlebells, but the friend's response was revealing: "You need to know more about kettlebells."

This simple observation triggered Shaun's characteristic thoroughness: "That's when I thought, okay, so let me find out a little bit more."

His research led him to Mike Mahler, who directed him to Pavel's RKC (Russian Kettlebell Certification) course in America. In 2004, Shaun and his wife made the journey to the United States for what would become a transformative experience.

The Baptism by Fire

Shaun's recounting of his first day at the RKC certification is both humorous and relatable to anyone who has experienced intensive physical training:

"First day I got back to the hotel, I said to my wife, 'That's it. We have wasted all our money coming here. I'm never going to pass this course.' I was sore, my hands could hardly close. I was tired. All I wanted to do was get some food and sleep."

I interject with my own similar experience from years later: "That was my first day in Seoul, South Korea, when I did mine in 2011. After the first day, I said, 'I don't know how I'm going to wake up tomorrow, how I'm going to pass this, I have no idea.' Got very little skin left on my hands, and Saturday morning I got up, and I don't think I had any muscle in my lower body that wasn't sore."

Shaun nods in recognition of this shared experience: "How did you feel after the end of the second day, though?"

"Much better," I admit.

"Exactly," Shaun confirms. "I went back and did the second day, but by the end of the second day, I was feeling so much better. Look, I was still tired, but I was feeling better. You can see the end of it now. By the end of the third day, I passed."

This experience brought Shaun a crucial revelation: "What I understood was that for a year of doing kettlebells, reading the book, and watching the video, my wife lied to me for that whole year because I looked nothing like Pavel. I couldn't do it the same. And I realised that in the first hour of the course, I had been playing with these, but not really understanding what they're there for and how to do the exercise properly."

The immersion in proper technique and coaching transformed Shaun's understanding: "What I learned on that weekend actually changed the direction I wanted to take my life in. That was the start of when I became a more professional instructor, professional coach."

Rather than immediately capitalising on his certification, Shaun spent several months refining his skills: "When I got back, after that weekend, I realised I'm not a coach yet. I know a few things, and a little more than others know. For about three, four months, I just trained family and friends for nothing, because if you pay nothing, you can't expect anything."

This humble approach – recognising the gap between certification and mastery – exemplifies Shaun's thoughtful approach to strength coaching. Only after this period of practice did he launch his business, "Kettlebells for Africa," and begin his professional coaching career.

The Beast Tamer Challenge

As our conversation shifts to specific achievements, I ask Shaun about a particular milestone in his strength journey – something that made him "the first" in the kettlebell world.

Shaun explains that in 2004, kettlebell training was still relatively new, with the heaviest bell being 32 kilograms (about 70 pounds). That year, they introduced a 48-kilogram bell (nearly 106 pounds) – a formidable weight that a petite woman on his staff can now demonstrate for perspective.

With the introduction of this massive kettlebell came a challenge: "They've got this thing called the Beast Tamer challenge. And if you could press it with one arm, you can pistol squat it – pistol squat means a one-leg squat – and you can do a tactical pull-up, which means overhand grip, pull from dead hang to bar against your neck, chin over the bar with this 48-kilogram kettlebell hanging on the chain. If you can do all three of those, you become the Beast Tamer."

The timing couldn't have been more challenging. Shaun spotted this announcement four weeks before he was scheduled to return to the U.S. to assist at another certification while his wife completed her own.

"I saw this and I needed something to train for," Shaun recalls. "So I said to her, this is what I'm going to do. But I had a problem. The heaviest bell I had was a 32-kilo bell. And I couldn't do one pistol squat yet."

When I ask how he overcame this "small problem," Shaun's response reveals the methodical approach that characterises his training philosophy:

"I put together a plan."

He used a Smith machine at progressively lower heights for the pistol squat, always working with his 32-kilogram bell since "there's no point in learning to do a pistol squat with a 16 if you're going to do it with a 48." He employed Pavel's "grease the groove" method – performing frequent, fresh reps throughout the day without ever training to failure.

Shaun loaded a barbell and practiced side presses for the press, working up to 65 kilograms. "Being on a bar, you've also control that rotation. So it really got the shoulders really nice and strong."

The pull-up training involved adding progressively more weight: "I did pull-ups, grease the groove style, pull-ups under a swinging bar. So I'd have two 16 kilos under the bar, I'd slide them onto my feet, pull up, go down, drop one, pull up, go down, drop the other, pull up, and down."

Throughout this compressed training block, Shaun maintained the principle of never pushing to the point of form breakdown: "The idea is that you never push the body to the point where you make the mistakes, you lose the form, and you injure yourself."

He supplemented this specific preparation with deadlifts for overall strength and visited a physiotherapist three times "just to open up the shoulders a little bit." Looking back, he acknowledges the intensity of this preparation: "It was probably 12 weeks of training condensed into four weeks... I wouldn't recommend that four-week condensed for most people out there, but it worked for me."

The tension builds as I ask whether he passed the challenge. Shaun explains that when they arrived the day before the course began, most of the assistants were seeing the 48-kilogram kettlebell for the first time: "We were unpacking and it was the very first time most of us had ever seen a 48-kilo bell and we're like, 'Wow, let's try this.'"

In this impromptu session, Shaun successfully pressed it and completed a pull-up, but he hadn't tried the pistol squat – "the first full pistol squat I had done was on the Sunday before. Sunday night we left."

When the official Beast Tamer challenge occurred during the course, Shaun found himself competing alongside Brett Jones, Senior Instructor, and Thomas Phillips, assistant instructor. "Thomas and Brett missed one of them, and I managed to get all three of them on that day. I have the privilege, the honor, of being the original Beast Tamer."

With justified pride, he adds, "Up to this day, I'm still the heaviest Beast Tamer. I did it at 116 kilos of body weight. Not the tallest anymore, but still the heaviest. And that was at the age of 35."

Making Time for What Matters

Shaun's achievement with the Beast Tamer Challenge exemplifies a core theme in his approach to strength – the power of consistent effort directed toward a clear goal. "The message from this is consistency. You will beat the odds. You had a plan. You went out every morning, put the effort in, and executed the plan. And that led to success. And don't let obstacles stand in your way."

This leads naturally to a discussion of one of the most common obstacles people face – the perception of not having enough time to train. When I mention how often I hear excuses about lack of time from clients, Shaun doesn't dismiss these challenges but offers practical wisdom from his own experience.

"Training for the Beast Tamer Challenge, I had obstacles," he acknowledges. "My very first obstacle was, I didn't have a 48. I had a 32. That's a big obstacle."

Beyond equipment limitations, Shaun was navigating significant personal and professional challenges. "We had four kids at home, and I was in the process of winding down two businesses," he explains. "These were very successful companies, but our contracts had been cancelled, forcing us to find different sources of income. It was an incredibly stressful period of my life."

Despite these circumstances, Shaun made training a priority: "I needed to focus on this and I made the time."

His advice is straightforward and actionable: "People say, 'I don't have time to train.' If you've got a little courage corner set up in your home, you can always start off half an hour earlier in the day. If you wake up at six, wake up at half past five and go do your training."

Shaun identifies a common pattern that derails many training plans: "If you leave your training to the end of the day, that's normally when things fall apart, because when you go to work, you plan to leave at five, crisis hits, you're there till seven. By the time you get home, you're stressed, you don't really want to train, it's getting late, kids, other responsibilities, and it's just easy to let that go."

According to Shaun, the solution is mental clarity and commitment: "The one thing that I learned is don't let those obstacles stand in your way. Decide what you want to do and then work towards that goal. And make the most of what you've got."

When I ask whether the rewards have been worth the effort, Shaun's answer is unequivocal: "Yes." He explains that achievements like the Beast Tamer Challenge are significant milestones but part of a larger journey: "It's a specialised goal. I think you need to have little goals along the way in your health, fitness, and strength training life. And that was my goal at that time."

His subsequent goal – "to become the best instructor and the best coach that I could be" – required the same commitment to personal practice: "To be a good coach, you need to internalise what you do so that you can teach it and you can help other people."

The Power of Example

The impact of Shaun's commitment extends far beyond his personal achievements. His children, now ranging from 16 years old and up, have all embraced some form of strength training. When I ask what role he played in their development, his answer is illuminating: "I think it was really just the role model. They see their parents get up in the morning, not only teach other people how to move and how to be strong, but practice it as well."

This modeling created an environment where his children absorbed proper movement patterns almost by osmosis: "I didn't have to teach them the technical side of doing a swing or the technicalities of doing a get-up. After years of just watching us, they were able to get in and do the stuff."

Shaun emphasises that introducing children to strength training should be driven by their interest, not parental agenda: "People always ask, 'What age should we let our children start training?' When they're interested. And that can be five years old. But don't make it a chore. Don't make it an effort. It must be fun."

The approach paid dividends – all of Shaun's children have excelled athletically: "My eldest son has just been selected for the South African Schools Under-18 A team for rugby. My three other children have all competed at a high level, too – my daughters played water polo, and my younger daughter competed at the provincial level. My youngest son also represented his province in water polo."

Beyond specific sports achievements, Shaun identifies two crucial elements that strength training has developed in his children: "The discipline of training, and discipline is about consistency. You do a little bit every day, and it adds up. It's like savings. You can't save by only putting money away once. But if you put a little bit away every day, at the end of the year you'll have quite a savings."

The Ferrari in the Garage

As our conversation shifts toward advice for men over 40 who are returning to exercise after years of inactivity, Shaun offers a vivid metaphor that perfectly captures the situation.

"We were all Ferraris in our day. We moved well when we were young. Then we parked the Ferrari in the garage for 20 years," he explains. "You are not going to take your Ferrari out and go 200 kilometres an hour down the drag unless you first check the tires, make sure that the bearings are okay, make sure there's oil, fill up with fuel, make sure your brakes are working, because you know when you go to 180 you need to stop as well."

This automotive analogy translates directly to the middle-aged body: "We've parked our Ferraris for 20 years, now we're getting in, now we're in our 40s, we think we need to do something about this. The first thing we've got to do is, are there any flat tires? That means, do we have mobility issues? Do we have ankles that actually move, hips that actually move?"

The process must be methodical: "A good coach will first check that. And I will first check. Can you move? How do you move before we start loading? So get you to move better. And once you're moving better, we'll get you to move stronger."

Shaun distills this approach into a simple progression: "Simple before complex, light before heavy, skill before load."

This perspective challenges common assumptions about fitness progress: "A lot of people confuse progression with load." He offers the example of ballet to illustrate his point: "If you look at a ballerina, a five-year-old dancing, looks good, does a pirouette, but it's not the same as a 23-year-old professional ballet dancer doing a pirouette. They're doing the same movement, but they're at a different skill level. The progression is not just in load, but it's actually in movement skill."

This insight runs counter to much of contemporary fitness culture. "This industry is so fixated on intensity and load," Shaun observes. "It's always about how much you can lift, how much you can bench, how fast you can run. But the real question should be how well can you perform these movements? And for how long can you sustain that quality?"

The dangers of prioritising intensity over quality are particularly acute for men returning to exercise after a long hiatus: "A lot of guys have parked their Ferrari in the garage for 20 years, and then they think they can immediately take it out and drive at 200 kilometres per hour," Shaun warns. "No, you can't. Your body isn't ready for that kind of stress after such a long break."

Even for those who have trained consistently, time brings changes that must be respected: "When I was 19 or 20 years old, I was benching 180 kilograms," Shaun reflects. "I can't bench that now—I'm close, but not quite there. If I tried to push myself to that level too quickly, I'd almost certainly injure myself. Our bodies change, and we need to respect that."

The psychological component is equally important in this process. "When you're coming back into training," Shaun advises, "don't fixate on what you used to be capable of doing. That was in the past. You'll inevitably feel like a failure if you constantly compare your current self to your former abilities. You'll never measure up to those memories, and you'll miss the opportunity to appreciate where you are now and the progress you're actually making."

The Road to Sustainable Strength

Throughout our conversation, Shaun returns repeatedly to the concept of sustainability – training to build strength for the long term rather than chasing short-term gains at the cost of injury or burnout.

This approach requires understanding the body's adaptation timelines: "Our muscles adapt quicker to load than our connective tissue and bone structure do. So our muscles can get stronger quicker."

For those unfamiliar with anatomy, Shaun clarifies: "Your connective tissue is around the joints. Your tendons, your ligaments." This explains a typical pattern Shaun sees among returning exercisers: "Many people complain of persistent aches in their joints—their elbows, shoulders, and hips. They describe a deep, underlying discomfort rather than sharp pain. This is very common, especially for those returning to training, and it's typically a sign that your connective tissue is being overstressed. Your body is telling you to slow down."

The consequences of ignoring these signals can be severe: "People don't tear biceps in the middle. They tear it at the origin/insertion. That's connective tissue. When we train, we need to allow the connective tissue to catch up in strength."

This principle applies to teenagers experiencing growth spurts and older adults returning to training: "We can look good, but ache inside. And that's not longevity. Eventually, you're going to stop. Eventually something's going to break."

As we conclude our exchange, Shaun offers to demonstrate two fundamental movements that epitomise his approach to building sustainable strength – the plank and the Turkish get-up.

What makes these exercises valuable, he explains, is that they train the body as an integrated system rather than isolated parts: "You want to be able to connect your feet with your shoulders, and all the way through. So you want to connect your left hip, right shoulder, and right hip to your left shoulder. You want to connect everything."

This connectivity provides the foundation for all movement: "That gives you stability, and enables you to move better and stronger. And move as a unit, not as a sum of individual pieces."

The Turkish get-up, in particular, represents a comprehensive movement education: "It covers almost every movement pattern that our bodies have. Push and a pull. Squat and a hinge. A lunge. A rotation. All in one."

"Swiss Army knife," I suggest.

"Exactly," Shaun agrees. "It's all there. Altogether. Learning how to connect everything together. And we only load once we're moving well."

This final statement perfectly encapsulates Shaun Cairns' philosophy – a thoughtful, progressive approach to strength that prioritises quality movement, respects the body's adaptation timeline, and builds capacity that lasts not just for a training cycle but for a lifetime. His journey from rugby fields to being the original Beast Tamer to coaching generations of athletes offers a model for sustainable strength development that serves men in their forties and beyond.

Reflection question

1. Shaun emphasises that "simple before complex, light before heavy, skill before load" should guide our training approach. How might you apply this philosophy to physical training and other areas of personal development in your life where you've been prioritising quantity and intensity over quality?

2. The Ferrari metaphor suggests that many of us try to perform at our peak without properly "checking the tires" first. What specific mobility issues or movement patterns might you need to address before adding significant load to your training, and how would improving these fundamentals change your approach?

3. Shaun demonstrates how consistent, everyday discipline—"a little bit every day adds up"—led to his achievements and his children's success through role modelling rather than forcing. What small, daily training habit could you implement that would be sustainable enough to practice consistently and potentially influence others around you?

EMBRACING DISCOMFORT: GEOFF WILSON'S JOURNEY INTO EXTRAORDINARY CHALLENGES

"Start small. Choose one minor challenge, face it directly, and overcome it completely. As you conquer these smaller obstacles, you'll build the confidence needed to tackle progressively larger challenges."
- **Geoff Wilson**

A Life of Adventure

The road winds up into the hills of the Gold Coast as I make my way to meet Geoff Wilson, veterinarian, world record holder, and polar explorer, preparing for perhaps the most ambitious expedition of his life. As I approach his property, the setting feels like a prelude to adventure – a sprawling hillside home surrounded by animals and overlooking the Australian landscape.

Geoff greets me with the easy confidence of someone accustomed to facing extraordinary challenges. In his late forties, he radiates energy and purpose that immediately contradicts the sedentary stereotype of middle age.

"My passion has always been just getting outdoors in whatever way, shape, or form, and also animals," Geoff explains as we settle in for conversation. "You can see from the house that we're surrounded by animals. The balance has kept it really fresh for me."

Despite approaching fifty, Geoff maintains the enthusiasm and drive of someone decades younger. "I'm in my late 40s now and I still mentally feel like I'm 24," he says. This mindset isn't just personal – it's something he actively promotes to others, particularly men his age.

"As I travel around Australia, particularly, there's an epidemic of men dying emotionally at 40 and then waiting till 80 to get buried," Geoff observes with genuine concern. This emotional death – the surrender to routine, comfort, and diminished expectations – is precisely what his life stands against.

His philosophy is deceptively simple but profound: "It's about pushing hard every day, and standing for your tribe, for your family, and making sure that you spend yourself up. You want to be buried at 80, knowing that you gave it your best every day."

This ethos of living fully and embracing challenge rather than comfort has shaped Geoff's remarkable life journey, which began in circumstances as extraordinary as the man himself.

From Uganda to Australia by Cessna

Geoff's adventurous spirit may be partly genetic, partly circumstantial – the product of a childhood that would seem like fiction if it weren't true. Born in Uganda in 1970 during the early part of Idi Amin's regime, his first years unfolded against a backdrop of increasing chaos and violence.

"My father was a veterinarian, as was his father and his father before him. So there's a whole line of veterinarians," Geoff explains. "He was working in Uganda at the time."

As political violence escalated, the Wilson family had a front-row seat to the country's descent into turmoil. "There was a river in front of our house," Geoff recalls, sharing his mother's description of those days. "There'd be a body a week, then a body a day, and then multiple bodies floating past the house. So the barometer on how Uganda was going was measured by how many bodies were floating past the house."

When the situation became untenable, the Wilson family made an extraordinary decision that would seem reckless if not for the greater danger of staying. "When it got to a point where it was obvious the country was going to fall apart, they decided to buy a light aircraft and fly all the way in a Cessna 175 to Townsville," Geoff explains.

The journey's audacity comes into focus as he describes it: "I was five, my sister was seven, and we jammed into this tiny tin box. And if anyone's seen a Cessna 175, they're tiny. Their cockpit is probably not much wider than a tiny car. And to fly that for 42 days with no support, it's just crazy."

The flight wasn't merely long – it was fraught with near-death experiences. "They had two times over the Saudi desert where the engine – they developed a ball of sand in the fuel tank for some reason – cut out twice. The plane fell for thousands of feet, the ball rolled away, and the engine restarted."

This harrowing journey, when Geoff was just five years old, established a template for his life – one defined by embracing rather than avoiding challenge and risk. "That was my first adventure, and I think it set the tone for the rest of my life," he reflects.

The pattern continues in his family today: "We have an adventure year and then a non-adventure year so the family can recover. And we're in the middle of an adventure year now."

The Antarctic Challenge

That "adventure year" Geoff mentions isn't just any adventure – it's perhaps the most extreme challenge he's ever undertaken. "I head off to Antarctica in nine weeks to do probably the most brutal campaign of my adventure career, which is an attempt to break the longest solo polar record. It's a journey of nearly 6,000 kilometers across Antarctica."

The scale of this undertaking is difficult to comprehend – a solo journey across the most inhospitable continent on Earth, covering a distance equivalent to traveling from New York to Los Angeles and back. And Geoff will attempt this alone, pulling heavy sleds, in temperatures that can plummet to -55°C (-67°F).

Preparation for such an extreme challenge requires physical conditioning and mental fortitude. "The mental side of solo polar travel is probably bigger than the physical side," Geoff notes. His typical traveling pattern pushes human endurance to its limits: "Up to 16 hours travelling a day, and then a bit of recovery, and then do it again. And it goes on for day after day."

This willingness to embrace discomfort rather than avoid it forms the core of Geoff's philosophy – not just for extreme adventurers but for everyone. "I think the other thing about these journeys is getting men, particularly, to understand that discomfort is not a bad thing. You need a little bit of discomfort in your life to keep you fresh and keep you strong."

He sees this principle as increasingly countercultural: "The whole world's way of everything becoming soft – it's not working. People elect for comfort over discomfort every time."

Yet Geoff carefully distinguishes between his specific challenges and the broader principle they represent. "I don't ever want people to look at what I do and go, 'If I'm not matching that standard, I'm not succeeding.' I really want them to go; they don't have to do a solo trip across Antarctica. Their adventure could be something a lot simpler, a lot lower key. But as long as they're getting off the sofa, that's all I'm interested in."

This democratisation of adventure – the idea that everyone can and should embrace some level of challenge and discomfort – makes Geoff's extreme journeys relevant even for those who will never set foot on polar ice.

World Records and the Boob Sled

Geoff's adventurous spirit has led him to accumulate several world records, each with a remarkable story. "They're all sort of bizarre endurance records," he says with characteristic understatement. "We held the longest kite journey on land for years," he begins, referring to an expedition using wind power to travel across land.

His list continues: "The first person to cross the Sahara Desert using wind power alone, and then we were the first team across from Australia to Papua New Guinea, kite surfing. And then so far, the longest solo polar journey by an Australian."

But perhaps his most unusual record involves what he calls "the boob sled" – a campaign that blended extreme adventure with a cause close to many Australians' hearts. "I did a journey about four or five years ago for the McGrath Foundation, and we made a sled out of Sarah's breasts," he explains, referring to a specially designed sled shaped like a pair of breasts to support the breast cancer awareness charity founded by cricketer Glenn McGrath after his wife Sarah's diagnosis.

"It was this crazy idea to make a sled shaped like a woman's breasts, and then drag that from one side of Antarctica to the other to raise funds for the McGrath Foundation," Geoff continues. What began as "a bit of a laugh" became a remarkable achievement when Geoff completed the journey in record time.

"That boob sled has gone all the way around the world, and the record has had nine men try and break it – the 53 days," he notes. This wasn't just any record – it had previously been held by one of Geoff's heroes, Norwegian explorer Bors Oosland (Børge Ousland). In a testament to Geoff's humility and strategic approach, he sought guidance from the man whose record he aimed to break.

"I contacted him and said, 'Listen, I want to break your record and I want you to train me.' And he was humble enough to go, 'Yeah, you're a bit crazy, but yeah, sure.'" Geoff laughs at the Norwegian's initial skepticism: "I don't think he really felt threatened by an Australian polar traveller. After all, what would we Australians know about polar conditions? We spend our lives on beaches!"

Despite this unlikely background, Geoff ultimately succeeded beyond anyone's expectations. "Eventually, I trained with people whom he trusted. And sometime later, I finished that journey in 53 days and took 14 days off his record."

This achievement is even more remarkable because subsequent attempts by better-funded and potentially stronger explorers have all failed to beat Geoff's time. "Since then, nine men have tried to break the record—men with better funding and possibly greater physical and mental strength than me. But I believe they lacked a deeper purpose for their journey. Several came within 24 hours of breaking my record, but none have succeeded."

The stakes of such extreme adventures are underscored by a sobering fact: "One guy died in the process. So it's a brutal, it's a brutal place."

Yet even this record-breaking journey wasn't Geoff's ultimate goal. "That record, eventually, will fall. It amazes me every year that it doesn't get beaten. But it's not the original journey that I wanted to do. The original journey I wanted to do was the longest solo. And that's the one we finally got the permission for."

His upcoming expedition – the 6,000-kilometer journey across Antarctica – represents the culmination of this long-held dream. "November fifth and sixth, step off the plane and be held accountable for what I've spoken out," he says, referring to his imminent departure date.

The Science of Extreme Endurance

To undertake a journey of such magnitude requires mental fortitude and precise scientific preparation. Geoff reveals the complex calculus of extreme endurance when I ask about his nutritional approach for the Antarctic expedition.

"It's really difficult because the food makes up half my weight," he explains. "So I have about 180 kilos of payload, and I just measured the food, I think it's 95 kilos."

The nutritional challenges are multifaceted: "The problem with it is if it's too high in fat, your bowel can't absorb it. But if it's too low in fat, it's too heavy." This requires careful balancing of macronutrients: "I'm getting about nine kilocalories per gram of fat and four and a half for carbohydrates."

Geoff's daily nutrition strategy has been refined through trial and error: "What I've found really works well for me is a very strong breakfast – thirteen to fifteen hundred kilocalories for breakfast."

This isn't ordinary breakfast food. Working with Brook Farm in Byron Bay, Geoff had specialised food developed specifically for his needs. "They made a granola and a porridge that came in at about seven or eight hundred calories in two hundred grams. And I returned it and said, 'Listen, it tastes great, but it's not high enough in calories. You need to get the calories up.'"

The solution was as innovative as it was intense: "They cooked it again under pressure and infused it with macadamia nut oil. So macadamia oil is one of the highest calorie natural oils we have, and it came back at 1,300 kilocalories, which is almost like drinking petrol."

Adapting to such calorie-dense food required a training regimen: "The first couple of times we ate it, it was like having a laxative. Like it's so rich in oil that you just turn into an animal and run and go find a hole in the snow." With characteristic humor, Geoff adds, "There aren't many toilets available where we train, so you're running out with a shovel and going, 'Shivers, this is bad.'"

Over two weeks, Geoff gradually increased his portion sizes until his body adapted. "By the end of the two weeks, your bowel is adjusted to absorbing that big hit in the morning."

His full daily nutrition plan is equally scientific: "With a combination of protein powder, sausage, and pure fat, such as butter. Over the full day, you're taking a big breakfast and then three small lunches every two hours. And then your evening meal is a big calorie hit as well."

Despite this careful planning, the math of polar expedition remains brutal: "It's about 6,000 kilocalories a day. Your bowel can't absorb any more than that. So that's the maximum. I'm burning about 9,000 calories a day."

The inevitable result is dramatic weight loss: "Over a 90-day journey, I'd expect to lose probably 25 kilos. So it's a brutal campaign. You come out looking like you've come out of Belsen or one of the concentration camps."

This physical deterioration must be managed carefully: "You don't want your body loss to be so rapid that you don't have the strength to pull the sleds. And that's the tricky thing with the journey of this length – is realising you're going to lose biomass, you can't, there's no way you can avoid it, but can you hold on long enough to get the journey done."

Geoff's previous expedition taught him hard lessons about this delicate balance. "During my last journey, I lost 22 kilos. I made several critical mistakes, including losing two weeks' worth of food supplies. By the final three days before pickup, I had absolutely nothing left to eat."

These final days without food were particularly devastating: "Your metabolic rate is absolutely burning. And then as soon as you start putting food in, you start getting cold and burning muscle, because you've got no fat left at that point."

These insights reveal the complex interplay between nutrition, metabolism, and physical capacity in extreme conditions. Geoff summarises the key factors for success in polar expeditions: "The nutrition side is fascinating, and it's one of three critical elements that determine success or failure on these journeys. If I had to rank them, I'd say your mental approach is first, nutrition is second, and your body's biomechanics is third. Get any of these wrong, and the expedition will likely fail."

The Four Legs of Antarctica

Geoff's approach to his Antarctic journey demonstrates the same strategic thinking that has made him successful in previous expeditions. Rather than viewing the 6,000-kilometer journey as a single overwhelming challenge, he has mentally divided it into four distinct segments.

"I've broken the journey into four legs," he explains. The first leg will take him "from the Antarctic coast all the way to the pole of inaccessibility, which is, it's basically if you drop the pin in the middle of Antarctica at the point that's furthest from any coast, so the hardest place to get to."

This destination has historical significance: "No Australian's ever been there. There's a statue of Lenin there that the Russians put there in 1958. So I'll go and have a hug with Lenin."

The first segment, covering about 1,100 kilometers, serves a specific strategic purpose: "That first leg is just getting bedded in, getting comfortable, testing the systems, not breaking anything."

The second leg continues from the pole of inaccessibility to the more famous South Pole – "another 800, 890, I think, to the South Pole." Geoff characterises this segment simply as "just a physicality. It's just an endurance event."

It's the third leg that Geoff identifies as the journey's most critical challenge: "The third leg is where this whole journey could either be a success or failure because it's a 1.3 kilometre vertical climb over 880 kilometres."

To put this in perspective, he breaks down the math: "If you think about that, for every 880 metres you go forward, it's about a metre and a half vertical ascent. Which doesn't sound like much, but pulling 150, 160 kilos – by then it'll be a significant climb."

This segment presents unique challenges beyond the physical strain: "All of our weather reporting indicates that there'll be very light wind or no wind, so it could be a lot of hauling. And the hauling in deep snow, you just can't physically pull 160 kilos."

The solution requires extra effort and strategic adaptation: "I'll have to split load, which split loading is where I'll split the sleds, pull one sled up three kilometers, ski back down, pick the second one up, do it again. So to cover three kilometers, you're skiing nine. And to do that for 880 kilometers."

Adding to the challenge are the extreme temperatures at this elevation: "Dome A is the coldest naturally occurring place on planet Earth. In January, it could get down to minus 45, minus 55. So the cold is a concern. Hands, feet, face. At that temperature, in an hour, you could get frostbite."

The visualisation of success on this third leg is particularly important to Geoff: "I'm already visualising my boot stepping on the top of Dome A over and over again. I know with certainty that I'll get there."

The fourth and final leg offers the reward of descent: "Once I get to the top of Dome A, then it's just staying safe and trying to keep my body weight up while I make the two and a half thousand kilometre run downhill back to the coast."

Geoff's preparation includes technical solutions for the unique challenges of the third leg – particularly the need to travel uphill against the wind while pulling heavy sleds: "One of the keys in New Zealand was setting up a kite system on really long lines, because the longer the lines, the better your upwind performance. And then the sleds set up like a catamaran rather than a monohull. So they're side by side."

This innovation proved successful in testing: "Amazingly, with that system fully loaded, I could do 45 degrees to the wind. This means that even if the wind is coming down Dome A, I can potentially tack uphill, which would be much quicker and less strain on the body than manhauling."

This detailed breakdown of the journey reveals Geoff's meticulous approach to extreme challenges – breaking seemingly impossible tasks into manageable segments, anticipating specific challenges, and developing strategies to address them before they arise.

The Lion Killer Approach

Beyond the technical aspects of his expeditions, Geoff has developed a philosophical framework that applies not just to polar adventures but to all of life's challenges. He calls it the "lion killer approach," and it encapsulates his mental strategy for facing adversity.

"I think that what I'd call the lion killer approach is really important," Geoff explains. "I talk a lot about this shift in mental attitude to lions in your life. So whatever your lion is, whether that's obesity, depression, anxiety, cancer, a child taking drugs within your family, marital stress, whatever it is, that's a lion coming into your life to destroy and kill."

This metaphor draws inspiration from an ancient biblical figure: "There's a Hebrew warrior named Benaiah whom I've always admired deeply. What makes him unique in historical records is that, unlike most warrior stories where men are commanded to fight, Benaiah chose a battle entirely of his own accord. He encountered a lion trapped in a pit while walking home from an official military campaign. No one ordered him to engage this threat—he made that decision himself."

The story continues with compelling details that make it particularly relevant: "The text specifically mentions it was a snowy day, adding to the harsh conditions. Benaiah was walking home after defeating two warriors in battle, so he was already physically exhausted. Despite this fatigue, he noticed a lion trapped in a pit—an aggressive predator, roaring and agitated by its confinement."

Rather than avoiding this threat, Benaiah takes an extraordinary action: "He jumps into the pit with no weapon and fights this lion with his bare hands and kills it."

For Geoff, this ancient story offers a blueprint for modern challenges: "I think modern-day life, we are taught to walk past. The lion is there, just walk quietly, maybe it won't kill you. It's the wrong approach."

Instead, he advocates a radically different response: "The shift in mental attitude I'm trying to convey is this: the last thing the lions in your life expect is for you to confront them directly—to grab them by the throat and squeeze the life out of them." This proactive confrontation of problems is particularly important for men in midlife: "For men, particularly to get through that 40 to 80 period and still be driven and energized, you cannot ignore the lions in your life. You need to deal with them."

Geoff suggests starting with smaller challenges to build confidence: "Start with the small lions. Like the little pussy cat in the corner. Jump on that thing, deal with it head-to-head. And then slowly your confidence in your lion killer approach improves to a point, then you've got the mental strength to do a solo for 90 days across Antarctica."

This mindset isn't innate but developed through practice: "That mental approach didn't start from me jumping in the pit with big lions. It started with little lions."

Geoff shares a compelling example from his expeditions with his son-in-law, Simon: "His first journey with me was crossing the Torres Strait. And 70 kilometres from the coast, he tapped out. He said, 'I'm done. I can't do this.' And I talked him through the rest of the journey, and he made it. But there was a point where mentally he was finished."

The transformation over time was remarkable: "Four years later, in Greenland, he's again partnering with me. And it was a brutal journey, probably five times the physicality of the Torres Strait journey. But at no point did he even think about tapping out. So his lion killer approach has been honed and developed over a four-year period."

For those feeling overwhelmed by their own challenges, Geoff offers encouraging advice: "If you're looking at your life thinking, 'I'm surrounded by lions everywhere and don't have the strength to face any of them,' here's my encouragement to you: Start small. Choose just one minor challenge, face it directly, and overcome it completely. As you conquer these smaller obstacles, you'll build the confidence needed to tackle progressively larger challenges. The key is to begin with deliberate action rather than passive avoidance."

Demanding a Change in Circumstance

This "lion killer approach" extends beyond merely facing challenges – it includes actively demanding better outcomes even when circumstances seem hopeless. Geoff illustrates this with a powerful story from his Greenland expedition.

"In Greenland, by the end of day seven, it looked as though we were not going to break any record other than the fastest team to starve to death in Greenland," he recalls. "We'd covered very little distance, we'd had terrible weather, less than 30 kilometers in a week."

His response to this discouraging situation was raw and physical: "I threw a man tantrum. I started punching the snow."

Geoff's answer revealed his refusal to accept defeat when his partner, Simon, asked what was wrong: "I'm not upset with you, you've been phenomenal, but I'm upset with the situation. We have trained harder than any duo I know has ever trained for Greenland. We've got the best sleds, best skis, best kites, best nutrition, everything, all the prep's been done. We should be conquering this, and we should be ahead of the game and on track for the record. I'm demanding a change in our circumstances."

What happened next seems almost mystical: "The next morning, we got up and the wind had shifted. And we put our boots on and in the next week we covered more distance than any pair has ever covered in the history of polar travel – over 1200 kilometers in a calendar week. And that set us up to break the record by over two weeks."

Geoff draws a broader life principle from this experience: "There's a point in time where you can demand a change in circumstance. And whether it's cancer, whether it's a failing business, a failing marriage – as men in your household, you have to stand."

This stance of determination and refusal to accept negative outcomes connects back to his lion killer metaphor: "It's about standing. It's about the Spartans in the gap saying, 'You shall not pass.' It's man after man in history who has gone, 'I'm going to change history here. I'm going to change circumstances.'"

The process begins with a decision: "It starts with you pounding the ground and going, 'No, I'm not going to see this happen the way that it's naturally happening. I want to change it.' And there's a supernatural shift that happens when you make that mental change and go, 'No, I'm not going to stand for this.'"

This philosophy – confronting problems directly, refusing to accept negative circumstances, and actively demanding better outcomes – forms the core of Geoff's approach to challenges of all kinds, from polar expeditions to everyday life problems.

As our conversation concludes, I realise that Geoff has already answered my planned final question about advice for men over forty looking to improve their health and fitness. His entire philosophy – embracing discomfort, confronting challenges directly, and refusing to accept limitation – provides a template for extreme adventurers and anyone seeking to live with greater purpose and vitality.

In an age where comfort is favoured and challenges are often avoided, Geoff Wilson stands as a reminder that our greatest fulfillment often comes not from ease but from the willingness to face difficulty head-on. His upcoming Antarctic expedition represents not just a personal quest for a world record but a living demonstration of the principles he advocates – facing the lion, demanding better outcomes, and refusing to accept the emotional death that claims so many men in middle age.

Geoff's parting message is clear: the principles remain the same whatever your personal "Antarctica" might be – whether a health goal, a relationship challenge, or a professional aspiration. Face it directly, prepare thoroughly, visualise success, and refuse to accept defeat. This is the path to achievement and a life fully lived.

Reflection Questions

1. What is your own "lion in the pit" that you've been walking past rather than confronting directly? Consider Geoff's "lion killer approach" and identify a challenge in your life—whether related to health, relationships, career, or personal growth—that you've been avoiding rather than facing head-on.

2. Where have you chosen comfort over growth in your life, and what would it look like to "demand a change in circumstance" as Geoff did in Greenland? Reflect on a situation where you've settled for disappointing results rather than standing firm and refusing to accept the status quo.

3. What would be your equivalent of a "small lion" that you could tackle first to build your confidence in facing larger challenges? As Geoff suggests, transformative change often begins with conquering manageable obstacles before taking on life's biggest challenges.

FINAL WORDS: THE ROAD AHEAD

You've reached the end of these pages, but this is far from the end of your journey. In fact, for many of you, this may be just the beginning.

Throughout this book, you've encountered wisdom from men who've dedicated their lives to understanding strength, health, and well-being. You've read stories of transformation—not just physical changes, but profound shifts in outlook, energy, and purpose. Perhaps most importantly, you've been presented with practical, actionable steps to guide your path forward.

But knowledge alone doesn't create change. Information without application remains merely potential energy.

The difference between the men who will close this book and continue as before and those who will use it as a catalyst for transformation lies not in ability, genetics, or circumstances—though these factors certainly play their part. The true difference lies in the decision. In commitment. In the quiet, powerful moment when a man says to himself, "This matters. I matter. And I'm ready to prove it through my actions."

That decision might seem daunting. After all, you have responsibilities, limitations, and decades of established habits. Work, family, and obligations already claim your time. Your body has its history of injuries, restrictions, and patterns. Your mind has its familiar doubts and comfortable rationalisations.

Yet consider this: the very constraints that seem to limit your potential for change—your age, your experience, your responsibilities—are precisely what give you advantages that younger men lack. You know yourself better. You understand value more deeply. You've learned what truly matters. And most importantly, you've developed resilience through facing life's inevitable challenges.

Remember that strength, health, and wellbeing at this stage of life aren't about comparison—neither to others nor to your younger self. They're about becoming the most vital, capable version of yourself today, and creating the foundation for how you'll live tomorrow. Progress isn't measured against an ideal, but in relation to where you started and your direction.

Every man featured in these pages faced obstacles. Every expert encountered setbacks. Every transformation story included moments of doubt, plateaus, and unexpected challenges. What united them wasn't extraordinary willpower or perfect circumstances—it was persistence and a refusal to let temporary struggles become permanent defeat.

As you move forward from these pages, carry with you not just information but possibility. The possibility that your body can still surprise you with its capacity for adaptation and improvement. The possibility that your mind can find new clarity and purpose. The possibility that your experience of daily life can be fundamentally transformed through intentional action.

Start where you are. Use what you have. Do what you can.

Perhaps you'll begin with small changes—walking daily, improving your sleep environment, adding strength training twice weekly, or simply becoming more mindful of what you eat and how it makes you feel. Perhaps you're ready for more substantial commitments. Either way, each step builds upon the last.

The road ahead has room for imperfection. For experimentation. For adapting approaches to fit your unique circumstances. There will be days of progress and days of maintenance. Days of breakthrough and days of rest. This isn't a sprint but a journey of sustainable change—one that accommodates the full complexity of a man's life while gradually shifting its foundations.

You've invested time in reading these words. Now I invite you to invest action in living them. Not because you should, but because you deserve the strength, vitality, and well-being that come from honoring your physical self. Because the people who count on you deserve your best. Because the years ahead hold possibilities that can only be fully realised through a body and mind operating at their potential.

The capacity for renewal doesn't diminish with age—it deepens with wisdom. Your best self isn't in the past. He's emerging right now, with every choice that prioritises your wellbeing, with every action that builds your strength, with every decision that honours the remarkable potential that still lies within you.

The final page of this book is merely the first page of what happens next.

What will you write with the life you have ahead?
The pen is in your hand.

www.ingramcontent.com/pod-product-compliance
Lightning Source LLC
Chambersburg PA
CBHW071709020426
42333CB00017B/2198